The Seriou...
to y...

John Byrne is a seriou... ...lly bits include lots of books for children and adults, comedy writing for TV and radio and his live 'stand-up cartoons' show. The serious bits happen when he mixes his comic talents with education work all over the world.

He lives in London with his wife, son and lots and lots of paper.

For Dr Miriam – now eat some proper food!

Text © 1997 John Byrne
Illustrations © 1997 John Byrne

Editorial: Amanda Li
Design: Donna Payne & Ali Myer

First published in Great Britain in 1997 by Mammoth
an imprint of Reed International Books Limited
Michelin House, 81 Fulham Road, London SW3 6RB
and Auckland, Melbourne, Singapore and Toronto.

The rights of John Byrne to be identified as the author and the illustrator of this work has been asserted by him in accordance with the Copyright, Designs and Patents Act 1988.

ISBN 0 7497 2944 9

A CIP catalogue record is available for this title from the British Library.

Printed and bound in Great Britain by Cox and Wyman Ltd, Reading, Berks.

This paperback is sold subject to the condition that it shall not, by way of trade or otherwise, be lent, resold, hired out, or otherwise circulated without the publisher's prior consent in any form of binding or cover other than that in which it is published and without a similar condition including this condition being imposed on the subsequent purchaser.

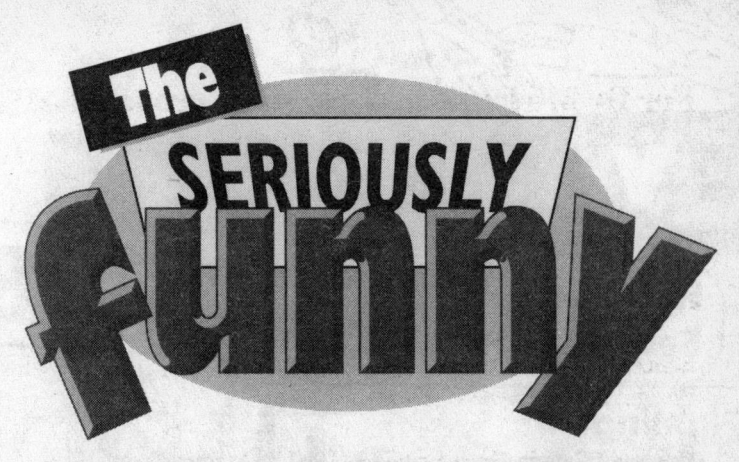

őt# The Seriously Funny Guide to your Body

Words, cartoons and jokes by

John Byrne

mammoth

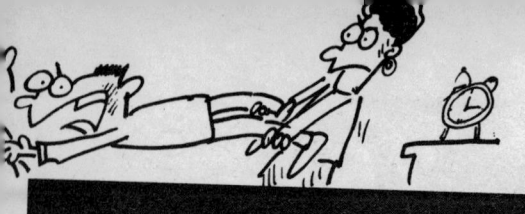

Vital Parts

How Much Do You Know About Your Body? 8
Test your physical and mental powers.

Fighting Fit 11
Food, fitness and mighty morphin'.

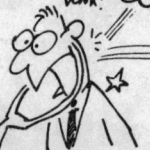

The Seriously Funny Workout 21
Excellent exercises to keep you in shape.

Seriously Sick 30
Help for hypochondriacs and sick jokes.

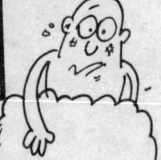

Looking Good 44
Everything from body language to beauty.

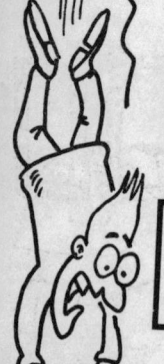

Dream On 56
What happens when you're fast asleep.

Face Up To It 68
Fascinating face facts!

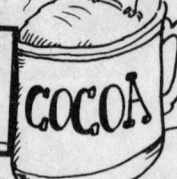

Body Bits 76
Your body parts get *their* say at last...

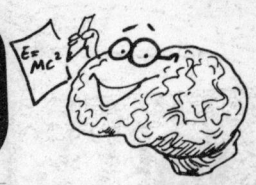

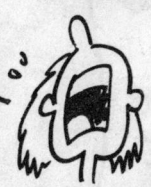

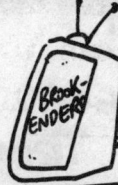

Young and Old 84
From babies to baldies, amazing age facts.

Tricky Tricks and Phenomenal Feats 92
Nifty tricks to impress your friends.

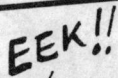

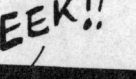

Mighty Molars 101
The tooth, the whole tooth and nothing but the tooth...

Problems, Problems 107
With Mr Funny as Agony Uncle, we've *all* got problems.

Your Toes to Head A to Z 118
An alphabet of things to do.

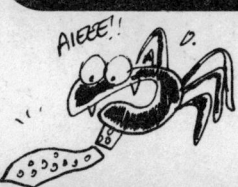

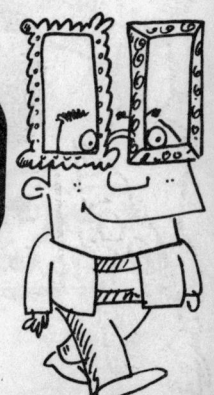

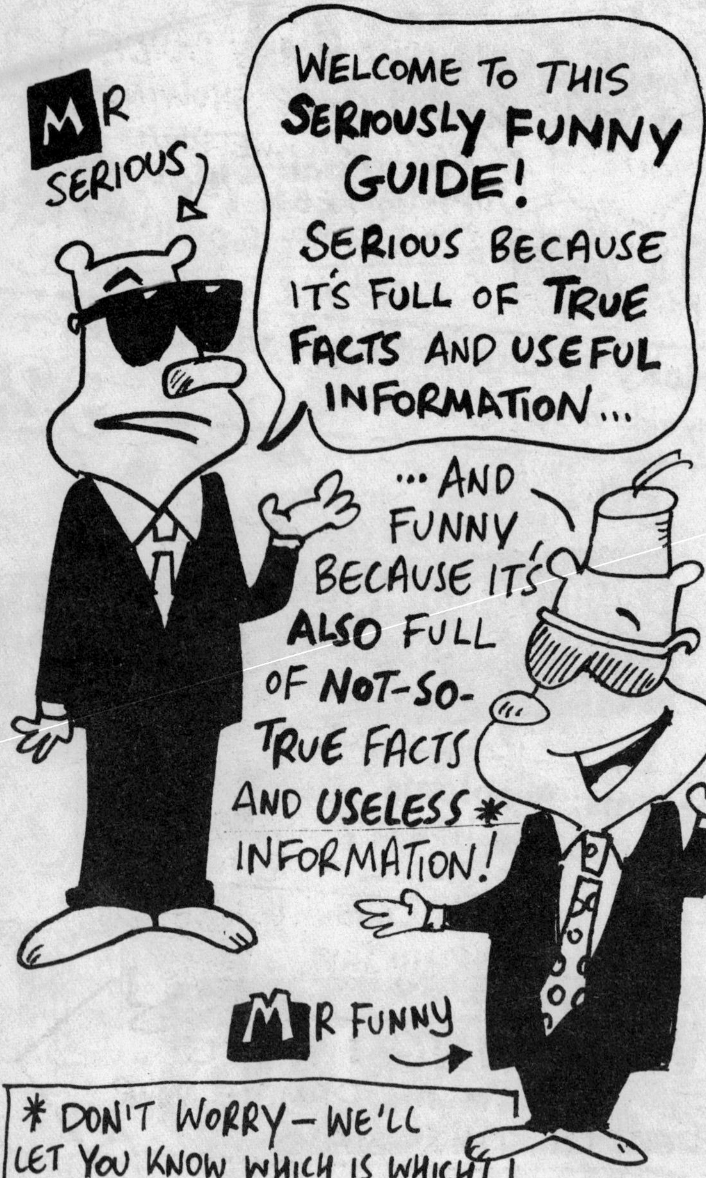
MR SERIOUS
WELCOME TO THIS SERIOUSLY FUNNY GUIDE! SERIOUS BECAUSE IT'S FULL OF TRUE FACTS AND USEFUL INFORMATION...
...AND FUNNY BECAUSE IT'S ALSO FULL OF NOT-SO-TRUE FACTS AND USELESS* INFORMATION!
MR FUNNY
* DON'T WORRY – WE'LL LET YOU KNOW WHICH IS WHICH!

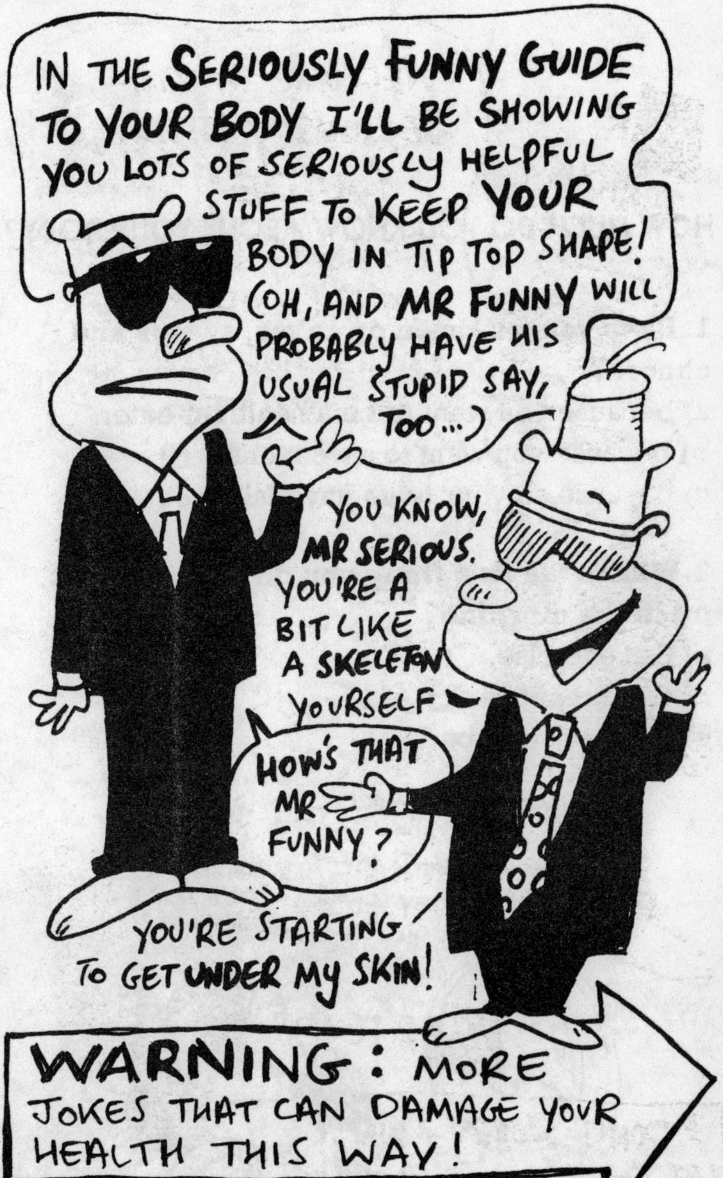
IN THE SERIOUSLY FUNNY GUIDE TO YOUR BODY I'LL BE SHOWING YOU LOTS OF SERIOUSLY HELPFUL STUFF TO KEEP YOUR BODY IN TIP TOP SHAPE! (OH, AND MR FUNNY WILL PROBABLY HAVE HIS USUAL STUPID SAY, TOO...)
YOU KNOW, MR SERIOUS. YOU'RE A BIT LIKE A SKELETON YOURSELF
HOW'S THAT MR FUNNY?
YOU'RE STARTING TO GET UNDER MY SKIN!
WARNING: MORE JOKES THAT CAN DAMAGE YOUR HEALTH THIS WAY!

QUIZ

HOW MUCH DO YOU KNOW ABOUT YOUR BODY?

1. Have you cut down on cakes, sweets and chocs...
a) because you want to be a healthier eater. ☐
b) because you want to save money. ☐
c) because all your teeth have fallen out. ☐

2. What's the first thing you do when you get up in the morning?
a) Get exercise. ☐
b) Get breakfast. ☐
c) Get back into bed. ☐

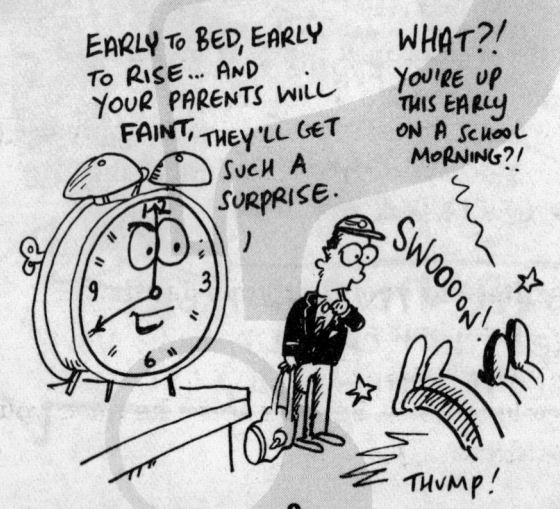

3. What's the proper amount of sleep needed for a healthy body?
a) Eight hours a night. ☐
b) Five hours a night. ☐
c) Sorry...I dozed off while you were asking the question. ☐

4. If you eat an apple a day it means...
a) The doctor is kept away. ☐
b) You'll soon get pretty bored with apples. ☐
c) There's a big security problem in the orchard. ☐

5. How often do you visit your dentist?
a) Every six months. ☐
b) Every two years. ☐
c) Every lunchtime. Bet he's sorry he gave you his home address. ☐

6. How would you describe your physical appearance?
a) Average. ❑
b) Attractive. ❑
c) Perfect. Good job I'm modest, too. ❑

7. How strong are you?
a) Quite strong. ❑
b) Very strong. ❑
c) Can't answer the question – the pen's too heavy. ❑

8. Which side of your brain do you use most often?
a) The right side. ❑
b) The left side. ❑
c) If I were using my brain, would I be doing this daft quiz? ❑

GOT ANY TIPS FOR STAYING HEALTHY, MR FUNNY?

YEAH – LET'S GET OFF THIS PAGE BEFORE THE READERS FIND OUT THAT THIS QUIZ HASN'T GOT ANY PROPER ANSWERS!

FIGHTING FIT
How Mighty Morphin' Are You?

What shape are YOU in today? Did you know your body shape falls into one of, or a combination of, three basic types: ectomorph, mesomorph or endomorph. Luckily, each of the three shapes can look great, so it's a shame that many of us waste time trying to make our bodies into something they're not. The most important thing is to be fit and healthy, and this book will give you lots of tips on ways to shape up and be happy with whatever shape you are!

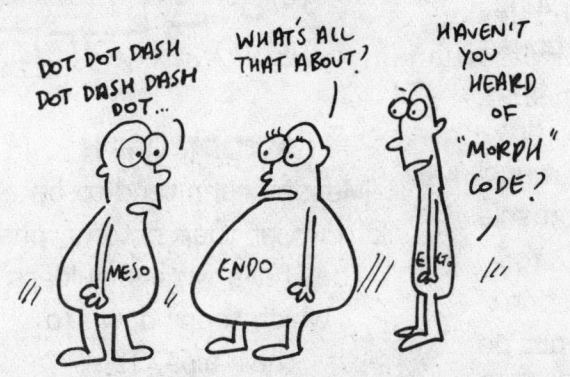

To help you find your body type, here's our handy guide. Of course, not everyone will fit a particular shape exactly – but you should be able to find a description which rings a bell. If you're still determined to find a new body shape, don't mess about with silly diets. Mr Funny has invented some brand new body types. So get morphin'!

Basic body shapes

ECTOMORPH

If you're an ectomorph, you're probably tall and lean with long bones and not much muscle. You don't put on weight very easily, no matter how much you eat.

ENDOMORPH

Endomorphs are short and naturally rounded. They are muscular and have wide hips and heavy bodies. They tend to put on weight easily.

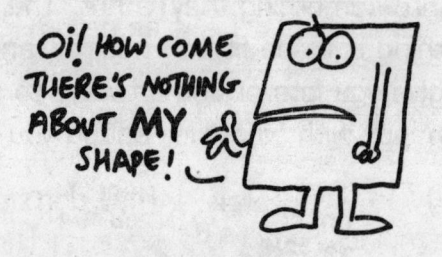

Oi! How come there's nothing about my shape!

MESOMORPH

Mesomorphs tend to be a lot curvier than ectomorphs. They have wide shoulders which taper down to their hips. They can be quite muscular, with medium to large bones. Like ectomorphs, they don't put on weight easily.

Mr Funny's body shapes

MESSO-MORPH
Messo-morphs are rumoured to be the same as mesomorphs but nobody can tell for sure, as their bedrooms are in such a state that no one's ever actually seen one.

TECHNO-MORPH
Techno-morphs are the same as ectomorphs only they aren't quite as tall because they spend most of their time bent over computer game consoles. They don't put on weight easily because they don't stop to eat unless they make it to Level Twelve. Techno-morphs don't worry much about finding clothes to suit their particular body shape as they don't come out of the bedroom very often.

EAST-ENDOMORPH
East-Endomorphs don't just have wide hips. They also have 36-inch screens on their TVs. They put on weight easily because they spend the whole day sitting around watching soap operas. There's one other important thing you need to know about East-Endomorphs – but you'll have to tune in next week to find out...

Mr Serious says: Be happy with whatever body shape you are. The morph the merrier!

THE BETTER BODY GUIDE

How to K.O. your B.O.!

WHAT HAPPENS

Sweating is good for you! It means your body is active and is cleaning out all its impurities. However, too much sweating can leave you dehydrated (lacking water) and when you are growing up can sometimes be a bit, well, smelly.

WHAT TO DO

The obvious way to beat B.O. (body odour) is to wash regularly – once in the morning and again in the evening, paying special attention to places like armpits and feet, which tend to sweat most. You can also use one of the many anti-perspirants and deodorants on the market, which will cut down on your sweating and cover up any smells. If your skin is especially sensitive, you may need to use gentler anti-perspirants without perfume (they still work!). You may also find that certain soaps dry your skin too much, so try to use ones which also have a moisturiser. Don't assume that the hotter your bath is, the cleaner you'll be – again, you may just dry your skin out. A warm bath will do the job just as well.

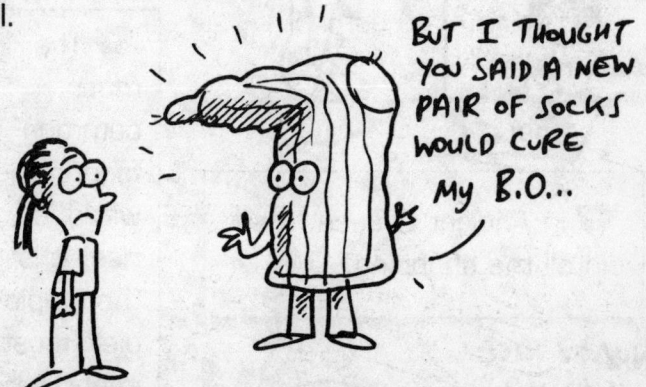

BUT I THOUGHT YOU SAID A NEW PAIR OF SOCKS WOULD CURE MY B.O...

Lastly, keep a good supply of clean socks, undies and t-shirts to change into as each one gets niffy. If you follow these simple guidelines, you'll be guaranteed that beating body odour is no sweat.

FUN FACTS

GET YOUR TEETH INTO THESE!

❗ Over 411,000 million gallons of water are drunk in the USA every day.

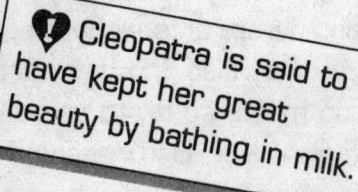

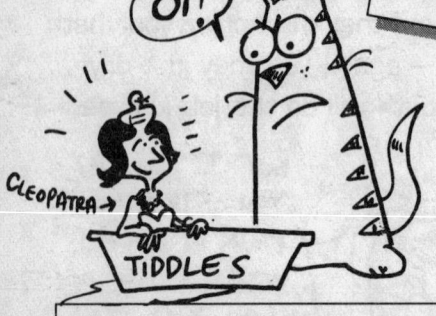

❗ Cleopatra is said to have kept her great beauty by bathing in milk.

Oi!

CLEOPATRA →
TIDDLES

❗ In Ancient Greece, men did all the shopping.

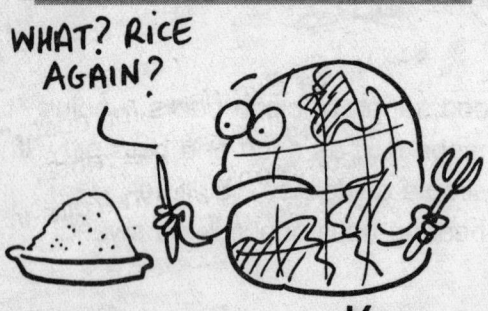

WHAT? RICE AGAIN?

❗ The most common food in the world is rice. It is the staple diet (most important basic food) of over half the world's population.

❤️ In many parts of the world, insects are a popular delicacy. They are also full of protein – but do wait until an expert tells you which sorts are okay to eat!

❤️ Shredded Wheat was the first ever breakfast cereal.

WOULDN'T YOU PREFER SOME SHREDDED WHEAT?

❤️ Babies have thousands more tastebuds then adults.

❤️ It was not until the nineteenth century that forks came into general use for eating. Until then most ordinary people used their fingers.

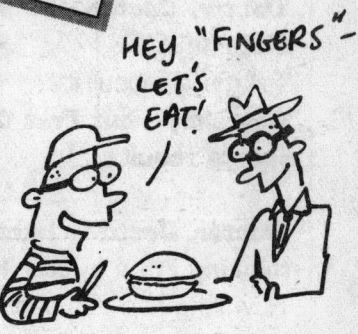

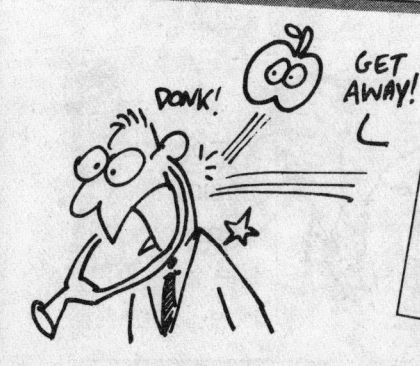

HEY "FINGERS" – LET'S EAT!

DONK!
GET AWAY!

❤️ Bad news for doctors – apples are the most commonly grown fruits in the world.

MEDICAL PRESCRIPTION

NAME: All kids everywhere

Laughter is the best medicine, so open wide!

'Doctor, Doctor – **I keep thinking I'm a wristwatch!'**
'It's nothing to get wound up about.'

'Doctor, Doctor – **I can't control my temper!'**
'How long have you had this problem?'
'Mind your own business!'

'Doctor, Doctor – **I keep thinking I'm Trevor McDonald.'**
'Tell me all about it.'
'Certainly – but first the sports results…'

'Doctor, Doctor – **I keep thinking I'm a butterfly.'**
'How long has this been going on?'
'Since I thought I was a caterpillar.'

'Doctor, Doctor – **I've got a very bad memory.'**
'We'll soon fix that.'
'We'll soon fix what?'

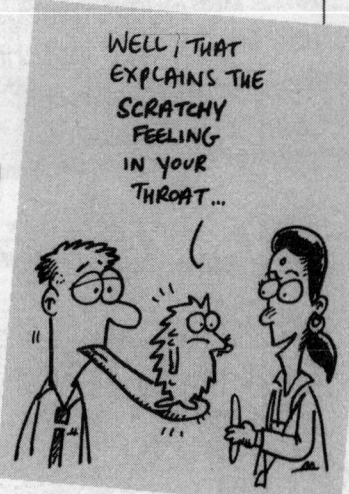

WELL, THAT EXPLAINS THE SCRATCHY FEELING IN YOUR THROAT…

BEWARE! JOKES AT LARGE

'Doctor, Doctor – I keep thinking I'm a D.J.'
'Stick out your tongue and say AHH.'
'I'm sorry, I don't do requests.'

'Doctor, Doctor – I think there's something strange about me.'
'Well, you look perfectly normal to me but please stick your tongue out.'
'Certainly – would you like me to stick it out of my right ear or my left ear?'

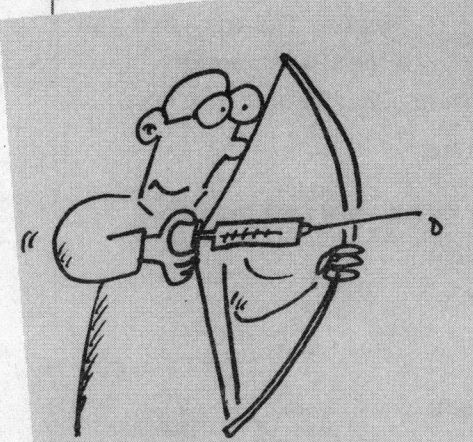

I WISH YOU'D GIVE ME AN INJECTION IN THE ARM LIKE EVERY OTHER DOCTOR!

'Thanks for curing me Doctor – I don't think I'm a cat any more. I'll gladly pay the £500...but isn't it a bit expensive for one hour's treatment?'
'It's only £20 for one hour's treatment. The other £480 is for the scratches all over my furniture.'

'*Doctor, Doctor* – I've been thinking I'm a tortoise since last November.'
'Good heavens – why didn't you come to me before now?'
'What, and come out of hibernation?'

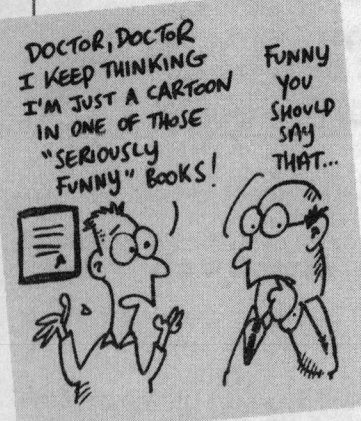

> DOCTOR, DOCTOR I KEEP THINKING I'M JUST A CARTOON IN ONE OF THOSE "SERIOUSLY FUNNY" BOOKS!
>
> FUNNY YOU SHOULD SAY THAT...

'*Doctor, Doctor* – I keep talking to myself.'
'I'll soon have you sorted out.'
'That's great, but would you mind not interrupting us while we're having a conversation?'

'*Doctor, Doctor* – I've got a very bad memory.'
'You certainly have – you were only in here five minutes ago.'

'*Doctor, Doctor* – I've got a very bad memory.'
'Haven't we done this joke?'
'Yes, but I wanted a second opinion.'

AND FINALLY...

Where do you send a rapper with a broken leg?
To the hip hop-spital.

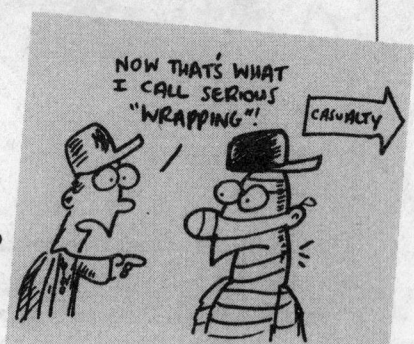

> NOW THAT'S WHAT I CALL SERIOUS "WRAPPING"!
>
> CASUALTY →

THE SERIOUSLY FUNNY WORKOUT

Warming Up

We all know that exercise is good for us – and it's fun, too! But before you start doing any sport or exercise routine you should always get your body ready. This is called warming up – and no, we don't mean wrapping yourself up in blankets and staying in bed all day.

Warming up loosens up your muscles and helps prevent you from injury. Follow these simple instructions and you shouldn't have to worry about aches and pains:

❶ Start off by walking around your room or on the spot. (Obviously this only applies if your room is tidy enough to walk around without spraining your ankle. Also, if you happen to have a dog called 'Spot' it's not a good idea to walk on top of him or you'll end up with some very nasty bite marks.)

❷ Stretch your arms above your head and you should feel your abdomen stretch. Pull your tummy in and your shoulders back. No need to do the hokey cokey or turn around.

❸ Now lift your knee and extend your leg. Lift each leg alternately for about two minutes.

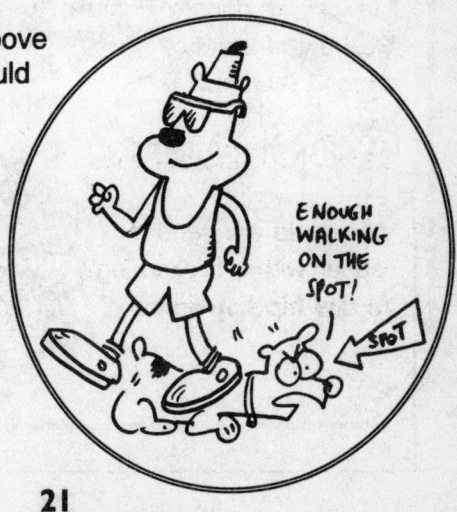

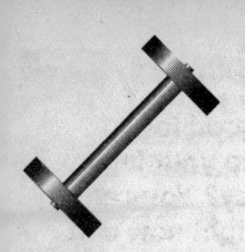

❹ Now kick your legs up to waist height. (One at a time, unless you fancy a sore bottom!) Keep going until your legs feel heavy.

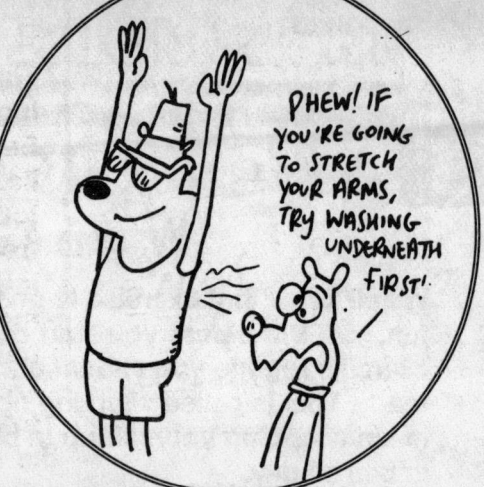

PHEW! IF YOU'RE GOING TO STRETCH YOUR ARMS, TRY WASHING UNDERNEATH FIRST!

❺ Finally jog around the room for a further two minutes and when you're finished, give your arms and hands a good shake.

Now you should be ready to try some of the easy exercises in this book. What do you mean you thought these WERE the easy exercises? Turn the page and get busy, you 'orrible little readers!

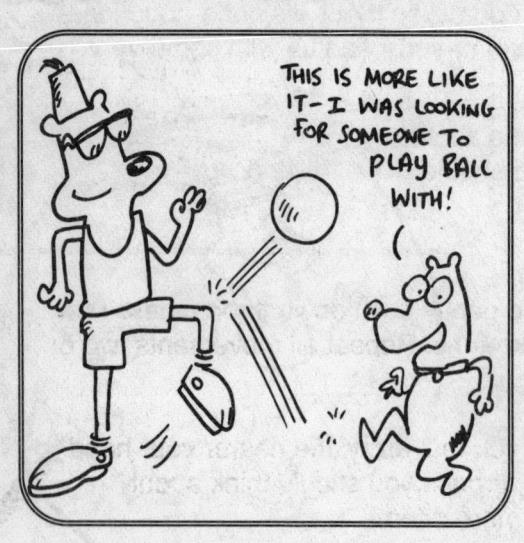

THIS IS MORE LIKE IT — I WAS LOOKING FOR SOMEONE TO PLAY BALL WITH!

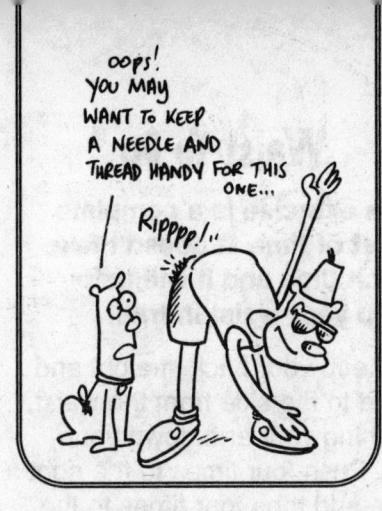

Toe Touches

These are good for loosening up your legs. Easy you say? You can bend over right now and touch the tips of your trainers? Very impressive – but you're meant to have your trainers ON.

Actually, you don't have to be able to reach all the way to your toes to do this exercise. Just stretch as far as you can and stop as soon as you feel any aches or pains. The more you practise, the further you'll be able to stretch.

❶ Stand up straight with your feet apart. Bending over, take your left hand over to your right foot (or as close as you can get it) and stretch up. Repeat with the other foot.

❷ Put both hands on the floor between your feet (or as far down as you can reach) and gently push down three times. Then stretch up with your arms. Repeat all movements two or three times.

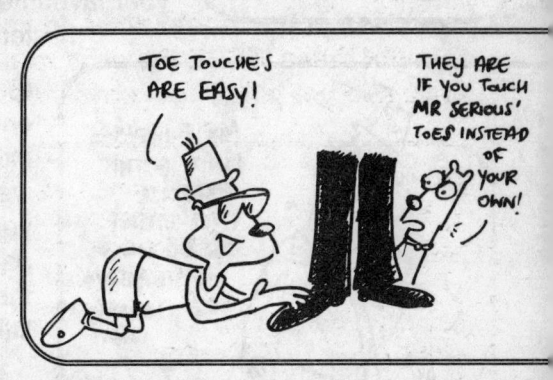

(Important note: If you feel dizzy, the nearer your head gets to your toes, perhaps you should think about washing your feet more often.)

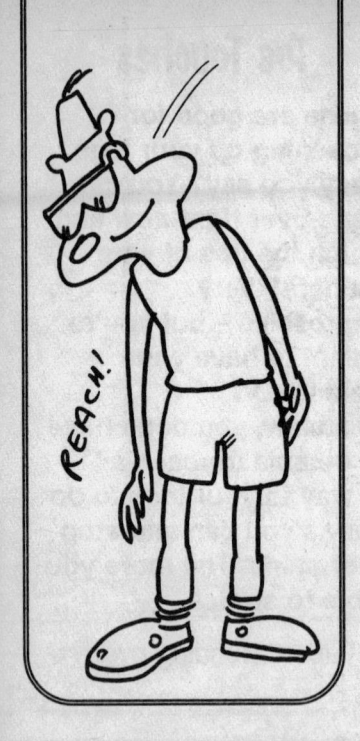

Waist To Go

This exercise is a complete waist of time. It doesn't take much time and it will help keep your waist in trim.

❶ Keep your back straight and bend to the side from the waist, pushing your arm down your leg. Push four times to the right side and then four times to the left side. Now push from side to side another eight times.

❷ It may encourage you to exercise if you do it in time to your favourite music on the stereo.

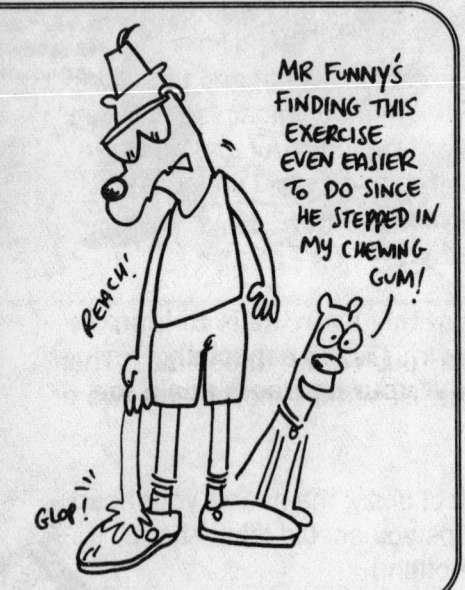

❸ It may *not* encourage you to exercise if someone walks in and sees you doing this particular exercise to the tune of 'I'm a little teapot...'

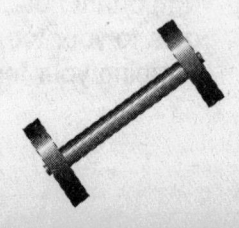

Jump To It

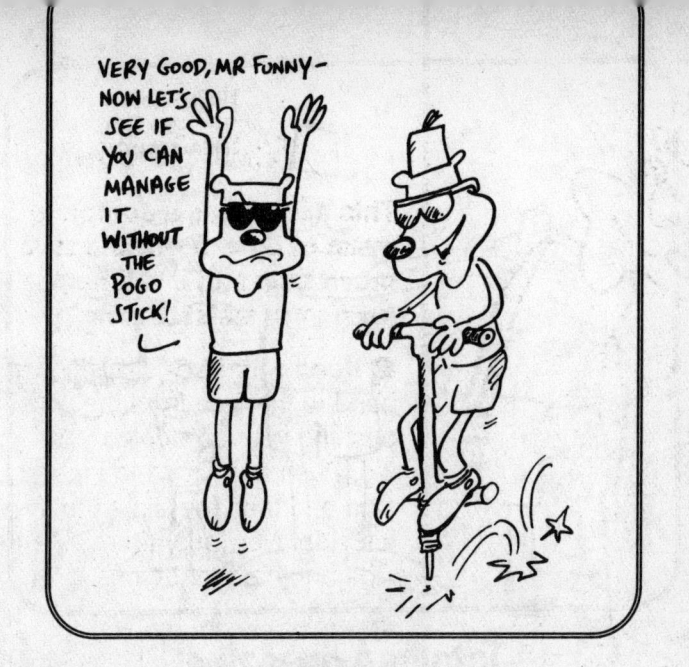

This jumping exercise is very easy and will help keep your thighs in trim.

Simply jump so that your feet are apart and then jump them back together again. Then try it again so that your arms go up in the air when you jump out and go down again as you jump in. Start off with eight jumps and increase the number as you get better.

IMPORTANT: The idea of this exercise is to jump in and out, not up and down. This is especially important to remember if your bedroom has a low ceiling.

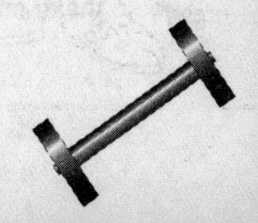

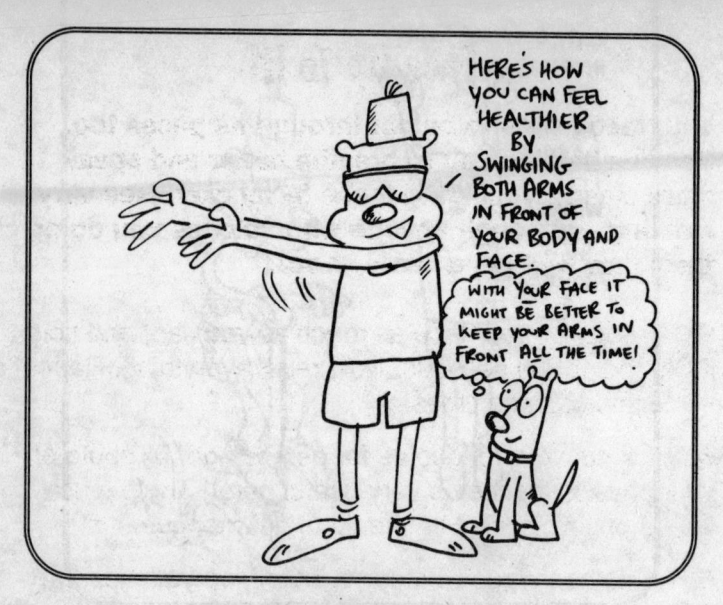

Totally Arm-azing!

Here's an exercise to loosen up your arms and shoulders:

❶ Swing your right arm around in a backwards circle from the shoulder.

❷ Now do the same with your left arm.

❸ Now do each arm in turn three times.

❹ Swing both arms in front of your face and body, five times to the right and five times to the left.

❺ Now swing both arms up and out five times.

❻ If you want to strengthen your arms, you can try this last bit with a tin of baked beans in each hand.

❼ If you don't want to have a lot of cleaning to do, you should make sure it's an unopened tin of beans.

Face Up To it!

Your face needs to be put through its paces too. Besides helping you to breathe better and speak more clearly, you'll find these facial exercises very relaxing – although anyone who catches you doing them may well get a nasty shock.

❶ Scrunch up your face as much as you can, and hold it like that for 30 seconds. Now relax everything. Repeat this exercise three times.

❷ Stick out your tongue as far as it will go. (A photo of your physics teacher is very useful here!) Try to touch the tip of your nose with the tip of your tongue.

❸ Try some tongue twisters to loosen up your lips. MR FUNNY FOUND A FINE FLOCK OF FOOLISH FANS FAKING FUNNY FACES might work, or try making up one of your own.

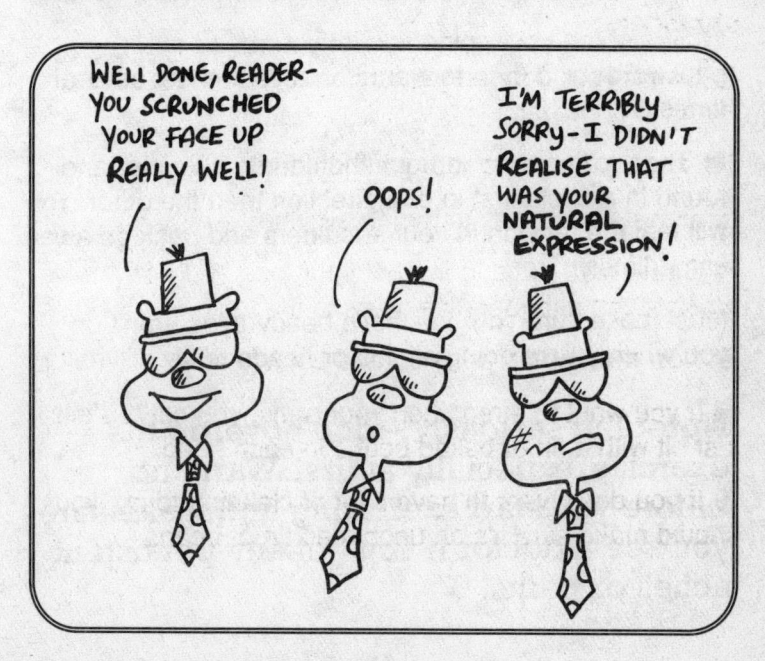

❹ Make sure you do these exercises in front of a mirror. If nothing else, you'll start the day off with a good laugh.

NOW THAT YOU'VE FINISHED YOUR EXERCISE ROUTINE, REMEMBER TO COOL DOWN. (No, that doesn't mean you can have a large dollop of ice cream on your cornflakes!) JOG GENTLY OR JUST WALK ON THE SPOT FOR A MINUTE OR TWO.

Oh, and here's one more simple exercise you can do at school...

Be a Desk Dynamo

YES! Just because you're at school doesn't mean you can escape the 'Seriously Funny Workout'. Besides, this is a great way to relieve stress and get your energy back even when you're trapped at your desk in the darkest depths of double history class.

❶ Straighten your spine and let your head roll backwards and then forwards onto your chest several times.

❷ Then roll your head from shoulder to shoulder and round in a circle first in one direction then the other. You will feel the tension in your shoulders and neck go away immediately.

(Just make sure your teacher's beady eyes aren't on you when you're doing all this or heads really will roll!.)

Note: But seriously – don't overdo the exercise, especially at first. Warm up before you start exercising and make sure you see a doctor if you get any persistent aches or pains.

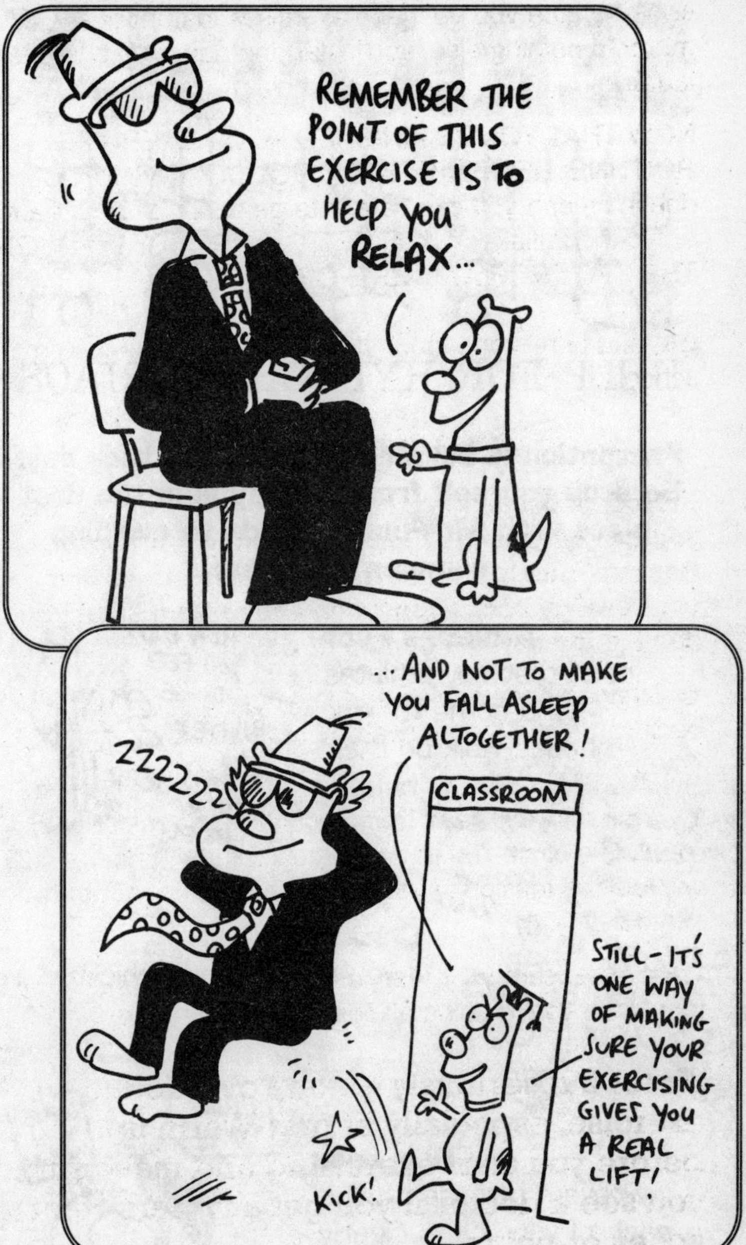
REMEMBER THE POINT OF THIS EXERCISE IS TO HELP YOU RELAX...
...AND NOT TO MAKE YOU FALL ASLEEP ALTOGETHER!
ZZZZZZ
CLASSROOM
STILL- IT'S ONE WAY OF MAKING SURE YOUR EXERCISING GIVES YOU A REAL LIFT!
KICK!

SERIOUSLY SICK

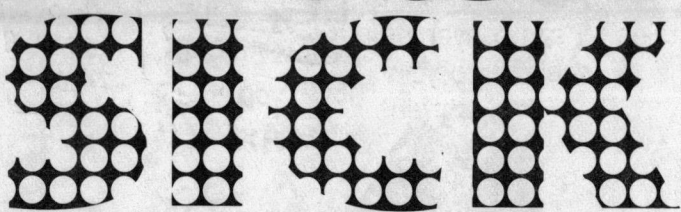

HELP FOR HYPOCHONDRIACS

Prevention is better than cure, so they say. So stop yourself from getting ill in the first place with Mr Funny's guide to avoiding common ailments:

Athlete's Foot
Insist that any athletes who come to your house walk on their hands.

How did you feel to be invited? I was head over heels!

Have you got chickenpox? No - I've got cock-a-doodle 'flu!

Chickenpox
If you see a spotty chicken...run!

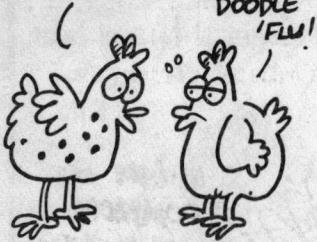

Hair Loss
Prevent hair loss. Label each of your hairs clearly.

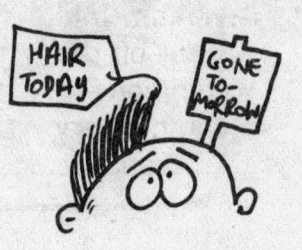

Hair today — Gone to-morrow

Food Poisoning
Keep a close eye on your food in case it tries to slip a cyanide tablet into your coffee.

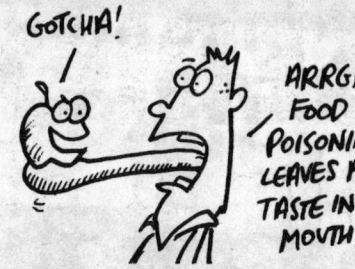

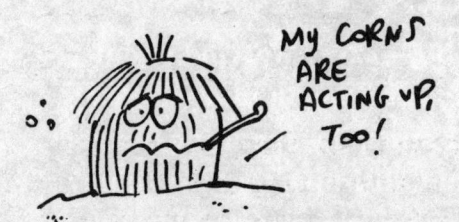

GOTCHA!

ARRGH! FOOD POISONING LEAVES A BAD TASTE IN THE MOUTH!

MY CORNS ARE ACTING UP, TOO!

Hay Fever
Make sure you take the temperature of your hay.

Running Nose
Don't let your nose run – hide its trainers.

READY, STEADY GLOW!

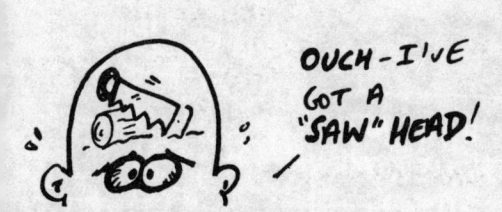

OUCH – I'VE GOT A "SAW" HEAD!

Splitting Headache
Instead of splitting your headaches, try to get them all over with at once.

Common Cold
Stay off the common – it can get very draughty.

*I MIGHT BE A **COMMON COLD**, BUT I'M NOT TO BE SNIFFED AT!*

Take Note!

Bothered by a big exam? Worried about outdoor training sessions in mid-winter? Why add to your stress by spending hours trying to forge that all-important sick note? Take advantage of modern technology as *The Seriously Funny Guide to Your Body* presents you with this handy all-purpose do-it-yourself version.

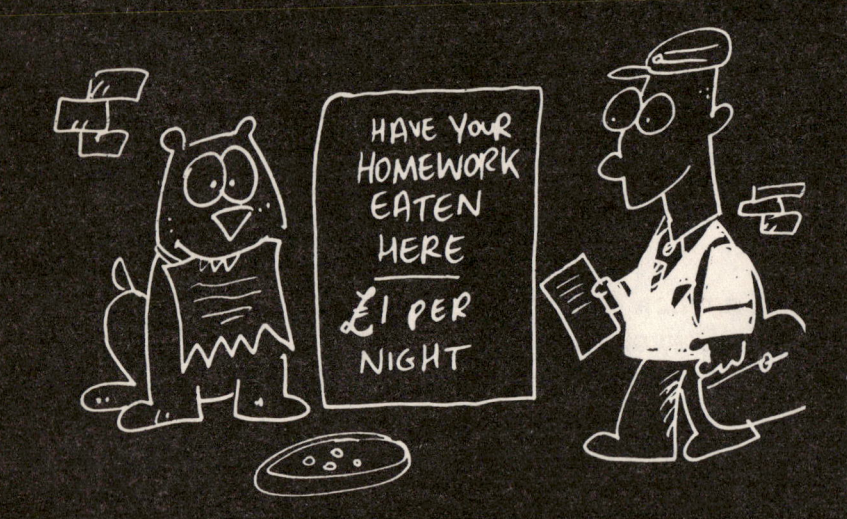

Dear
- ❏ Physics teacher
- ❏ Maths teacher
- ❏ Games teacher

**Please excuse ....
(insert name) from:**
- ❏ lessons.
- ❏ homework.
- ❏ detention.

As she/he has:
- ❏ a sore head.
- ❏ a sore stomach.
- ❏ a sore need to go the cinema.

She/he has also broken out in:
- ❏ red and blue spots.
- ❏ purple and yellow blotches.
- ❏ the colours of the school football team.

The doctor has recommended:
- ❏ a long stay in bed.
- ❏ lots of comics.
- ❏ a diet of burgers, chips and ice cream.
- ❏ talking as little as possible*

*this bit applies to teachers, not pupils.

However please note that in the unlikely event of a school trip to:
- ❏ EuroDisney
- ❏ Wembley
- ❏ Planet Hollywood

the patient may suddenly make a full and unexpected recovery.

Signed *My Mum.*

THE SERIOUSLY FUNNY FREE THERMOMETER

How many times has the school nurse held the thermometer in front of you and said 'SEE? 98.4 degrees – you're perfectly normal.' But you're not. Your temperature's shot up a few degrees because you're embarrassed – she might realise you have no idea what she's talking about. To avoid confusion, cut out and keep this handy guide to common temperatures and what they actually mean.

A The point at which water boils (the time it takes to reach this point gets longer and longer depending on how desperate you are for a cup of tea).

B Warm glow you get when you score the winning goal for your team.

C How hot under the collar you get when your goal is disallowed.

D How hot under the collar you get when the goal was allowed – but it was an own goal.

E How flushed you get over your favourite pop star.

F How flushed you get when people discover how flushed you get over your favourite pop star.

G The point at which water freezes (in other words the standard temperature of the school central heating pipes).

H How cold it is before you decide to stay in bed instead of going to school.

I Bone-chilling look from your mum when she discovers you in bed and not at school.

J How cold the school custard is.

K The chills you get down your spine when you realise the only dessert left is school custard.

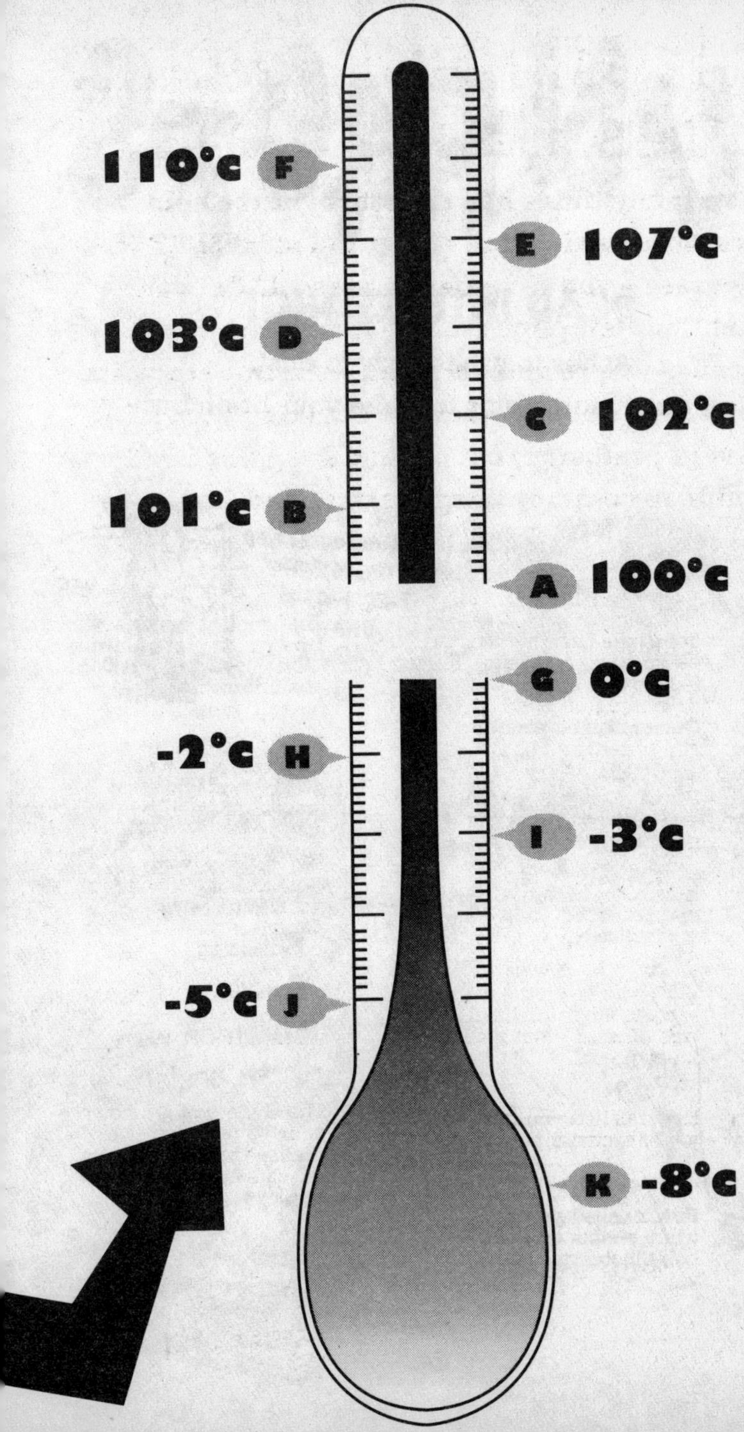
110°c F
E 107°c
103°c D
C 102°c
101°c B
A 100°c
G 0°c
-2°c H
I -3°c
-5°c J
K -8°c

FUN FACTS

DEAD INTERESTING!

Ashes to ashes, dust to dust,
Here are funeral facts to make your brain bust!

❣ The fourteenth century plague known as The Black Death took the lives of 75 million people – but only six people died in the Great Fire of London.

AS FAR AS I'M CONCERNED THE GREAT FIRE WAS A DAMP SQUIB! — DEATH

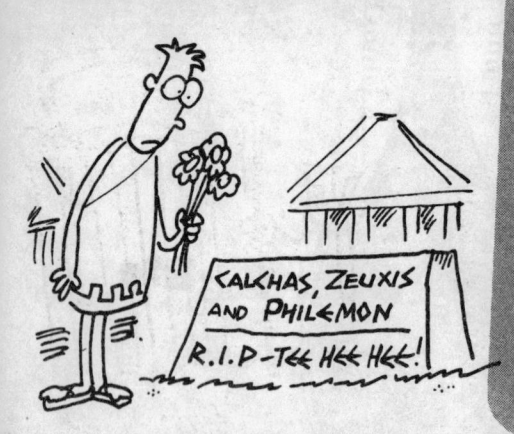

❣ Be careful when reading your *Seriously Funny Guides* – Calchas, Zeuxis and Philemon were three ancient Greek wise men who are said to have died from laughing.

CALCHAS, ZEUXIS AND PHILEMON
R.I.P-TEE HEE HEE!

💔 A survey in America showed that more people died in January and February than any other month. The months with the lowest number of deaths were July, August and September.

HE GOT OVER-EXCITED AT THE NEW YEAR PARTY!

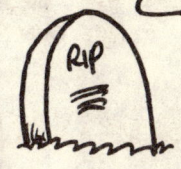

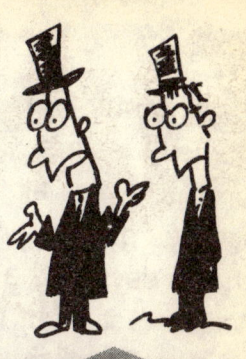

💔 Rasputin, the 'Mad Monk' of Russia, was eventually killed by his enemies – but only after they had poisoned him, beaten him with an iron bar and shot him twice. He was finally drowned.

IT'S BAD ENOUGH TRYING TO KILL A MONK IN THE FIRST PLACE – BUT SOME PEOPLE ARE MAKING IT A HABIT!

💔 Pope Stephen II had the shortest reign of any Pope. He was elected on March 24th in the year 752 and died only two days later.

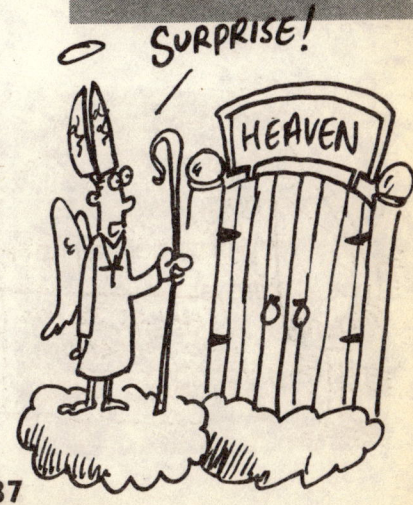

SURPRISE!

❗ Wyatt Earp, Doc Holliday and Frank James (Jesse's brother) were all famous gunfighters in the days of the Wild West – but none of them died in gunfights.

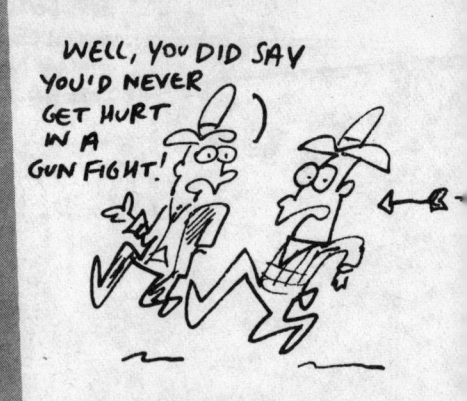

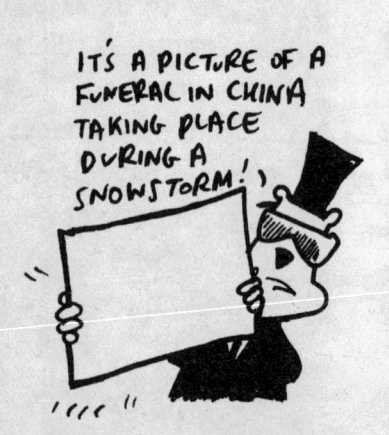

WELL, YOU DID SAY YOU'D NEVER GET HURT IN A GUN FIGHT!

IT'S A PICTURE OF A FUNERAL IN CHINA TAKING PLACE DURING A SNOWSTORM!

❗ In China, the colour worn at funerals is not black, but white.

❗ Geoffrey Chaucer, author of *The Canterbury Tales*, was the very first person to be buried at Poet's Corner in Westminster Abbey, London.

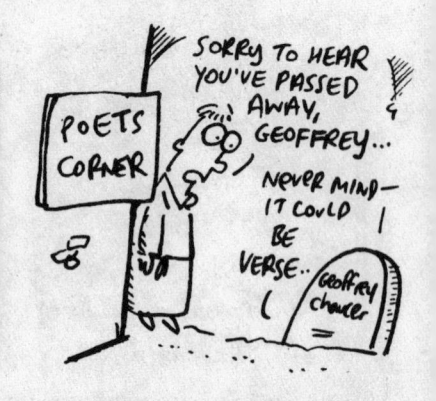

POETS CORNER

SORRY TO HEAR YOU'VE PASSED AWAY, GEOFFREY... NEVER MIND — IT COULD BE VERSE..

Geoffrey Chaucer

Why pay a fortune in medical bills?

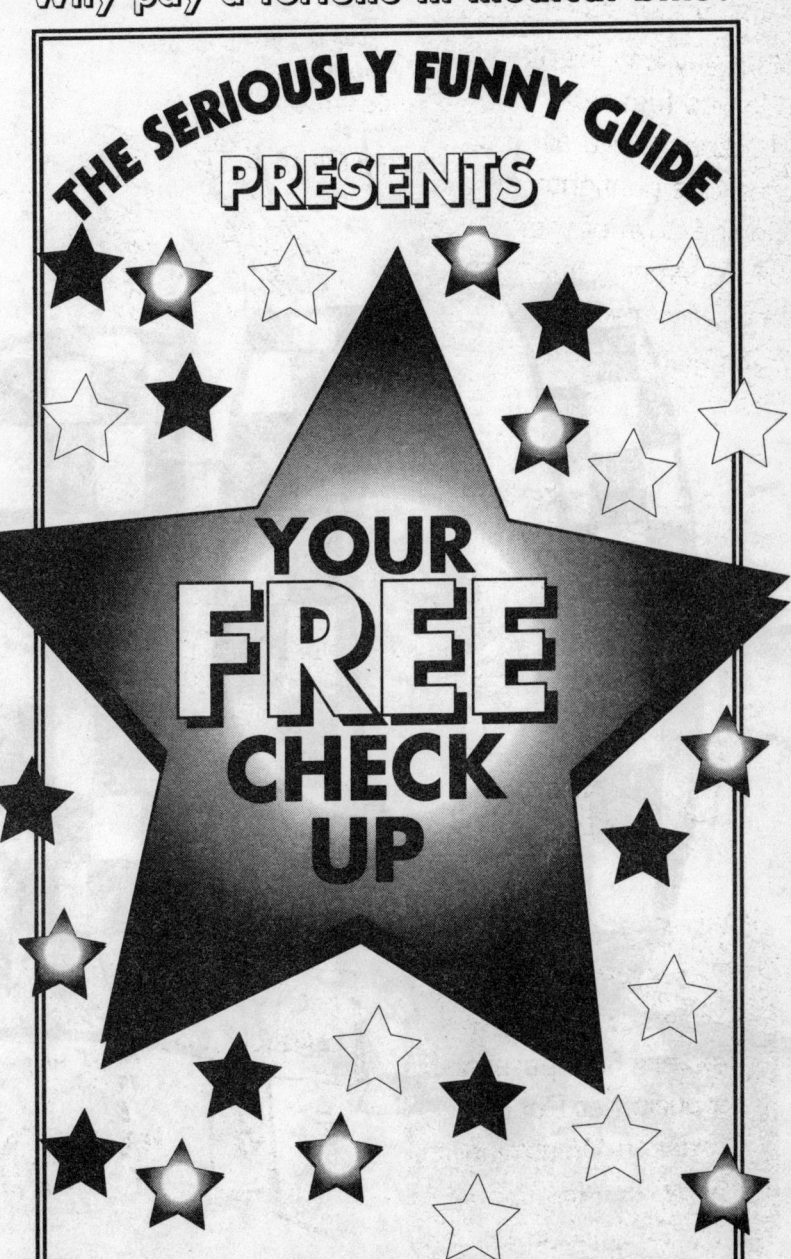

THE SERIOUSLY FUNNY GUIDE PRESENTS

YOUR FREE CHECK UP

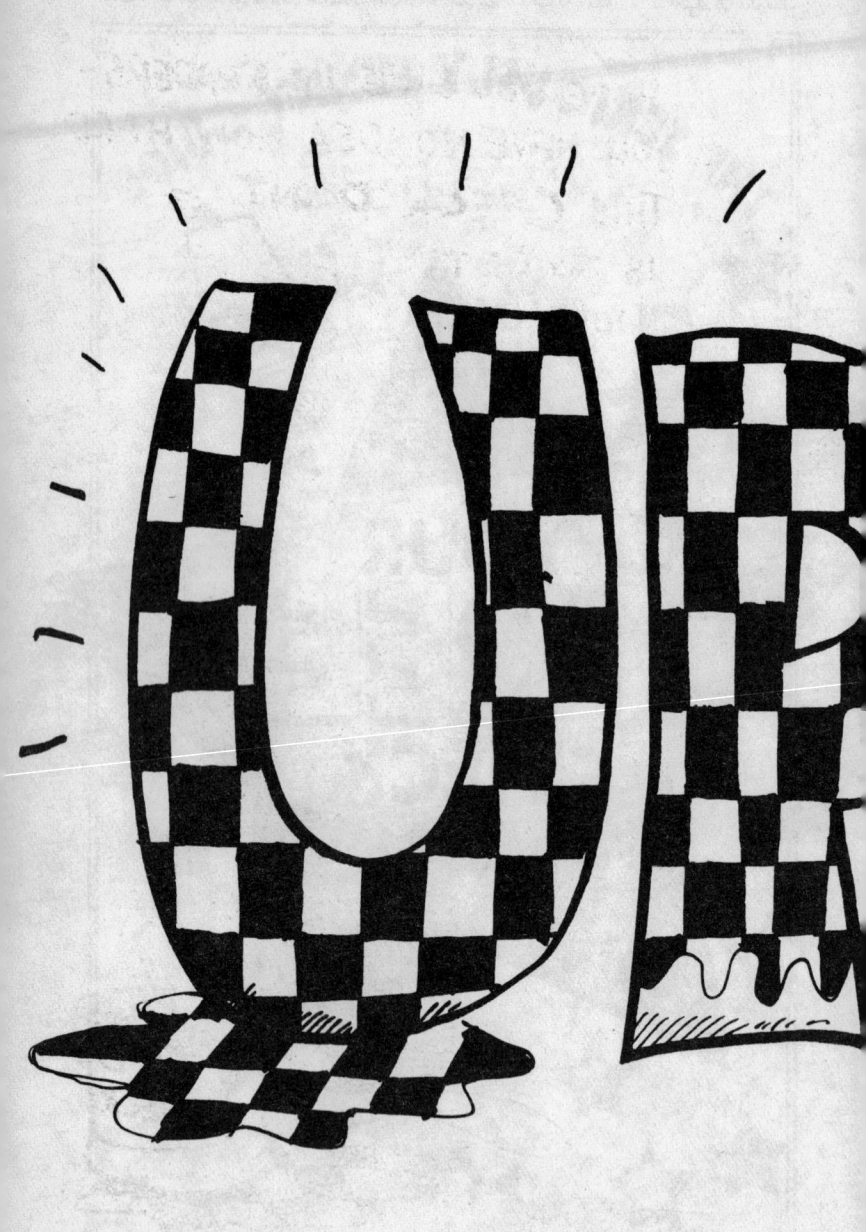

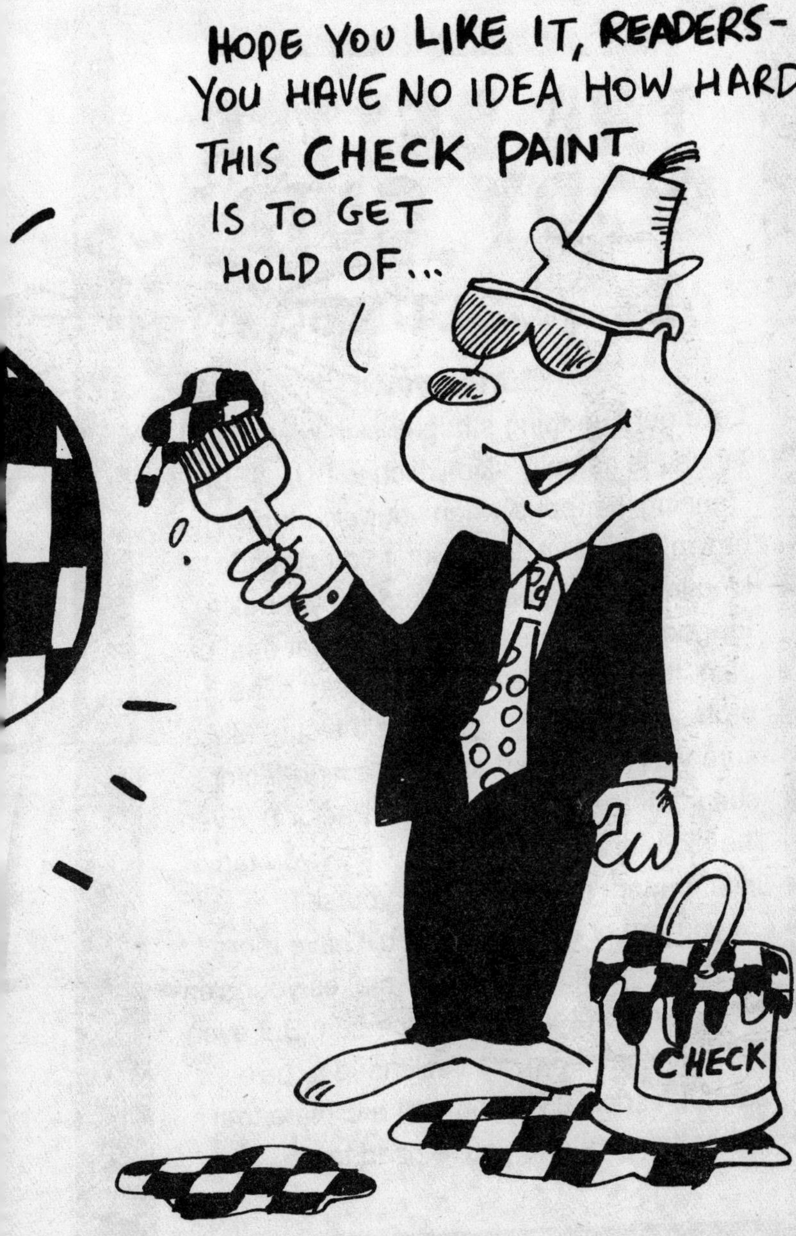
HOPE YOU LIKE IT, READERS- YOU HAVE NO IDEA HOW HARD THIS CHECK PAINT IS TO GET HOLD OF...
CHECK

THE BETTER BODY GUIDE

How to survive SUNBURN

WHAT HAPPENS

Let's get one thing straight: skin which is tanned is actually skin which is BURNED. 'Tanning' happens when your skin turns brown to protect itself. But if you stay too long in the sun you can damage your skin for good and cause yourself a great deal of pain. If your skin is fair, you'll need extra protection when you're out in the sun. Make sure you wear a hat and use a high-factor sun screen – never less than Factor 8. Even the high-factor sun creams will let you tan a little, but not enough to hurt yourself.

If you've got darker skin you'll have more melanin, the substance that makes your skin brown and protects it from the sun. But even dark skin can burn. You still need to be careful, especially if you visit a climate that's hotter than the one you're used to.

WHAT TO DO

Try not to get burned in the first place. Use sun creams and protections – and don't forget to re-apply the creams every two hours as your sweat will wash them away. If you really must go for that 'Baywatch' tan, try one of the many fake tans on the market.

But what can you do if the worst happens and you end up getting burnt? By the time you realise you're burning it's usually too late to turn back the clock. Here's what to do if this happens:

❶ Cover up, put on sunblock and get out of the sun immediately.
❷ Drink lots of water to prevent dehydration.
❸ Take a cool shower to lower your temperature.
❹ Apply after-sun cream or lotion.
❺ If the burning is really bad, see your doctor or go to the casualty unit of your local hospital immediately.
❻ Say to yourself: 'I will NEVER, NEVER, NEVER do anything this stupid again.'

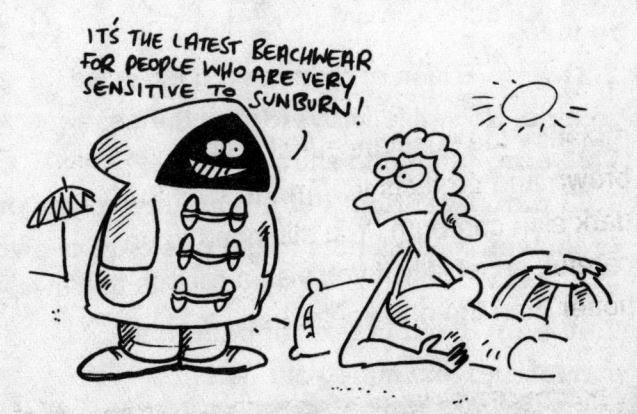

LOOKING GOOD

Mr Funny's Guide to Personal Grooming in Thirty Minutes

This health and beauty advice is all very well, but how do you get time to look your best in the whirlwind of everyday life? Never fear – Mr Funny is here to show you how.

10 p.m. Set the alarm for 6 a.m. in the morning. It's important to get up early.

6 a.m. Start the day with a good stretch. In other words, stretch your arm out and throw the alarm clock out of the window. It's also important to get some beauty sleep.

7.30 a.m. Get out of bed. Begin early morning exercise routine.

I'M OFF FOR MY BEAUTY SLEEP. I'M SURE YOU'D LIKE YOUR BEAST SLEEP AS WELL!

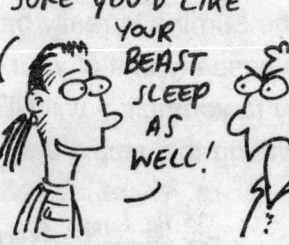

7.31 a.m. Finish early morning exercise routine. No sense in overdoing things.

7.32 a.m. Jump into shower.

7.33 a.m. Next-door neighbour throws you out of shower. Make a note to get one of your own, some day.

7.40 a.m. Stand in front of bathroom mirror and examine your face.

Jump back in horror as you realise you look a complete wally!

7.41 a.m. Breathe a sigh of relief as you realise it isn't the bathroom mirror after all – it's the TV and you've been looking at a breakfast TV presenter.

7.45 a.m. Brush your teeth.

7.47 a.m. Brush your granny's teeth. Now pop them in an envelope and post them back to her. How thoughtful!

7.50 a.m. Iron your clothes for the day.

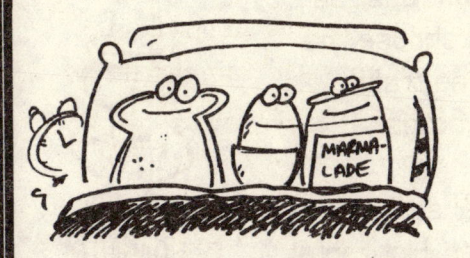

LOOK! BREAKFAST IN BED!

7.55 a.m. Iron your clothes again – this time remember to take them off first.

7.59 a.m. Whether you're off to school or work, you're ready to face the world, spotlessly clean, well-groomed and immaculately dressed. Not one detail has been forgotten.

8.00 a.m. Well, perhaps just one detail. Ruffle your hair, grit your teeth and tear your clothes to shreds as you realise this is Sunday morning and you've got out of bed for nothing!

Monsieur Funny's Fashion Tips

What good is having a bee-yoo-tiful body if you don't show it off properly? And who better to protect you from designer disasters and prêt-à-porter pitfalls than the stunningly stylish Mr Funny? Here are some well-known fashion rules – with Mr Funny's extra tips to help you.

❶ Bright colours always attract attention. Just be sure you don't choose the same colours as traffic lights or pillar boxes.

❷ Thin vertical stripes make you look thinner. Horizontal stripes make you look fatter. Black stripes on yellow mean you are looking at an escaped tiger.

❸ Clothes which are too tight make movement difficult. Especially when you and your friend try to wear something at the same time.

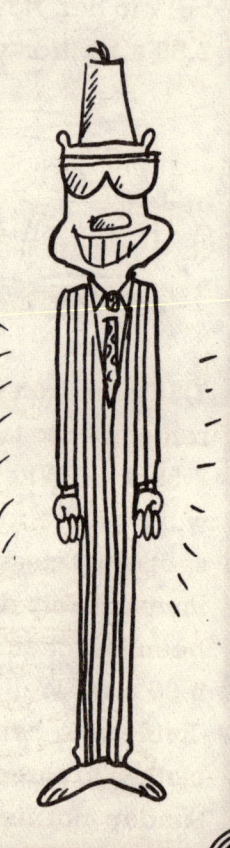

❹ Baggy clothes are good for wearing to discos. Just make sure the clothes aren't so baggy you never actually find your way to the dance floor.

❺ Always choose your shoes to match your clothes. (This can take some time as it's hard to find shoes which look like small shirts and jackets.)

❻ Shoulder pads are good for making your shoulders look bigger. You can get an even wider effect by wearing the clothes while they are still on the hanger.

❼ You can find great-looking old clothes in charity and bargain shops. Just make sure you choose the ones from the racks not off the backs of the people who work in the shop!

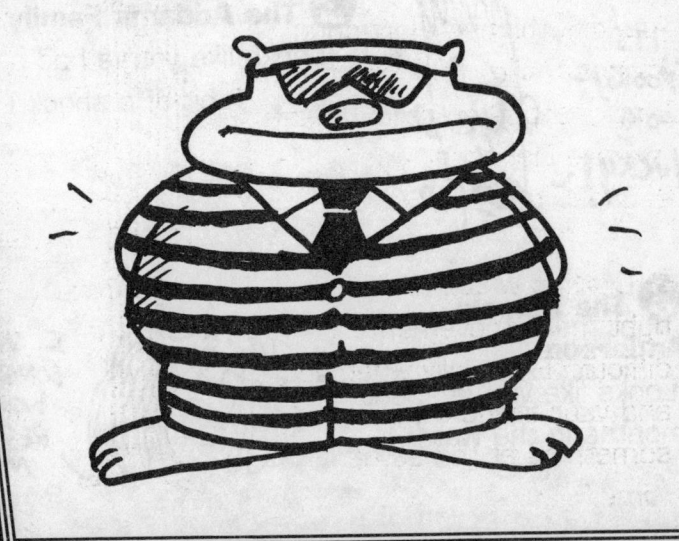

Hair We Go! Hair We Go! Hair We Go!

When your hair looks good, you feel like a real celebrity. But don't worry – even if you've had a real hairdressing disaster, you can STILL look like a star!

❶ The Jim Carrey
(So bad you have to wear a mask.)

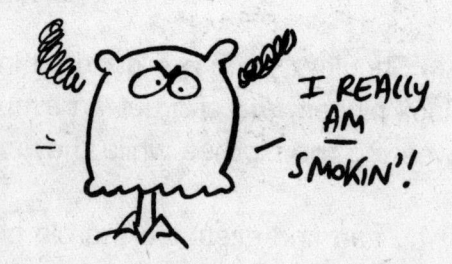

I REALLY AM SMOKIN'!

❷ The Addams Family
(Looks like you've had a bit of a shock.)

IT'S spooky-ooky-yucky!

❸ The Pamela Anderson
(Looks like you've spent months in the water.)

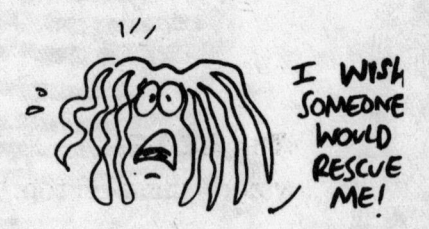

I WISH SOMEONE WOULD RESCUE ME!

4 The Mr Spock
('It's hair, Jim, but not as we know it.')

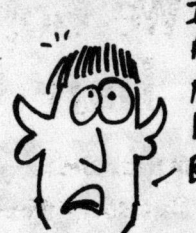

I'M MAKING A POINT OF NOT GOING BACK TO THAT BARBER AGAIN!

HAIRDRESSER I WON'T BE BACK!

5 The Arnold Schwarzenegger
(It looks awful but no one will dare tell you.)

WAHHHHH!

6 The Gazza
(So bad, you'll burst into tears.)

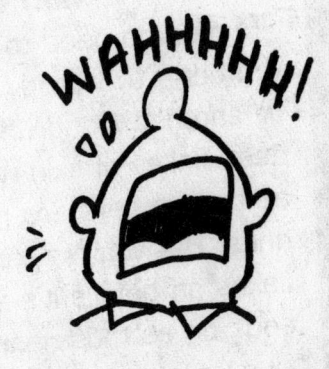

7 The Bugs Bunny
(You're having a bad hare day.)

8 The R2-D2
(Shiny and round on top.)

NOW THERE'S A HAIRCUT THAT REALLY IS OUT OF THIS WORLD!

THE BETTER BODY GUIDE

How to deal with DANDRUFF

WHAT CAUSES IT?

There's no need to let dandruff flake you out – everybody gets it at some time or another. Dandruff flakes are actually dead flakes of skin which fall off naturally as the old cells are replaced by new ones. But you may find that the skin flakes off before it's supposed to – and ends up as those annoying white spots all over your shoulders. This is particularly common as you enter your teens and your body begins to change. Dandruff can also be caused by not rinsing the shampoo out properly when you are washing your hair, causing a dry scalp. It's also thought that it may be stress related. Does your scalp get particularly dry and itchy around exam time?

WHAT TO DO

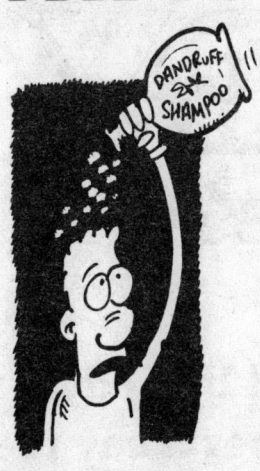

Not all of the medicated or anti-dandruff shampoos in your local supermarket may sort out the problem. In fact some of them are so strong they might just dry out your scalp even more. You may want to ask your doctor or chemist to recommend a good shampoo you can use. Follow the instructions on the label and remember you can do just as much damage by washing your hair too much as by washing it too little.

Try to relax more and see if that helps, and while you're waiting for the problem to go away, wear lighter-coloured tops which won't show the dandruff up so much.

Try not to scratch your scalp, no matter how badly it itches, as this will make it worse. You should also never share anyone else's brushes or combs.

If your dandruff is really bad, check with your doctor that it's not something different such as psoriasis. (Don't worry if it is – once you know what the problem is, it can be treated.)

Whatever you do, don't let dandruff get you down. If you follow these simple tips, the problem should be hair today and gone tomorrow.

BAFFLED BY BODY LANGUAGE?

Are you baffled by body language? The experts say that the way you stand, sit and generally move about is a guide to how you really feel about a situation or a person. Well, our resident expert, Mr Funny, has his own ideas about body language. Here's his handy guide to leave you really speechless:

❶ If the person you're talking to is tapping one foot, they are bored. (If they are tapping both feet, your personal stereo is too loud.)

❷ Don't always assume that if a person refuses to look you in the eye, they are dishonest. In some cultures it is a mark of respect to lower your eyes when you are talking to someone. (Then again, you may just have a face like the back of a bus.)

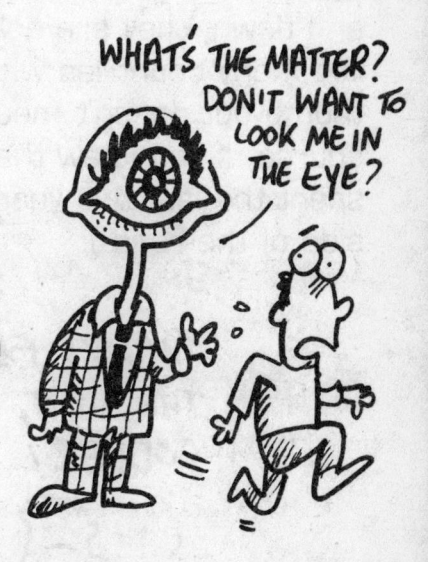

❸ When a person's pupils get wider, they are interested in what you are saying. (When a school teacher's pupils get wider, they are not interested in what the teacher is saying. They are interested in second helpings of school dinner.)

4 When a person puts their thumb out they are saying 'I want a lift'. (Don't stop unless you've got a car!)

5 When a person waves their hand up and down, they are asking for a lift in one of the many countries where putting your thumb out doesn't mean 'I want a lift'. (Of course, if you knew that you wouldn't have spent the last two years standing by the side of the road.)

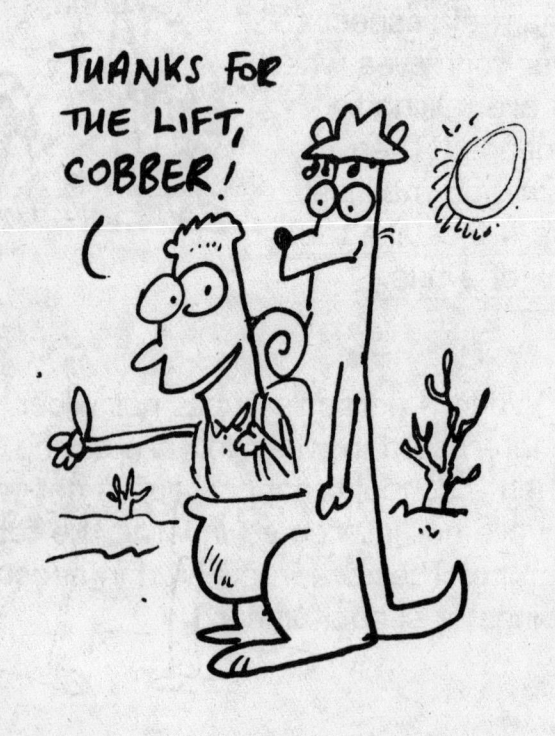

❻ If the person you are talking to makes nodding gestures and has a friendly expression they are enjoying the conversation. (Or else there's a television directly behind you.)

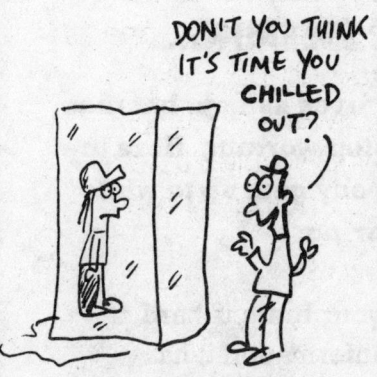

❼ If the person you're talking to has a glazed expression, they are not enjoying the conversation. (Or they are encased in a block of ice.)

❽ If the person you're talking to has no expression at all, you're standing on the wrong side of them, you fool.

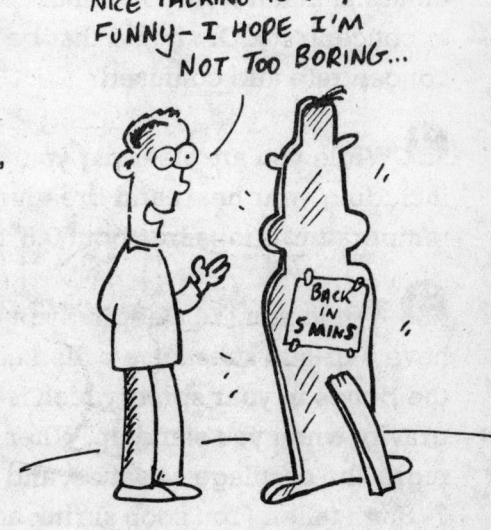

DREAM ON

WHILE YOU ARE SLEEPING...

We spend one third of our lives asleep, but that doesn't mean our bodies stop working. Here are some of the things your body gets up to while you're snoring:

❶ While you are sleeping, your brain is hard at work sorting through all the information it has received during the day. This is a very important job, as without it, your brain would be full of so many thoughts that it would become confused and unable to concentrate. Or should that be unable to concentrate and confused?

❷ While you are sleeping your body slows down – including your heart and breathing rates. Your body temperature drops by about $0.5°$ c.

❸ While you are sleeping you GROW TALLER. You have a gristly substance called cartilage between the bones in your spine, which is squeezed by gravity when you stand up. When you lie down at night, the cartilage expands, and you get about 7- 8mm taller. (You soon shrink again next morning.)

4 While you are sleeping you snore. (This might not be news to people who have to share the house with you!) Snores are caused by air rushing in and out of your nose and throat and rattling a flap of skin called the 'soft palate'. Some people snore all the time, others only once in a while. If someone complains about your snoring, remind them that some of the loudest snorers ever have managed to drown out the sounds of cars and trains passing by!

5 It's quite common to talk and walk in your sleep once in a while. Usually the talk is meaningless mumbling and sleep walkers wake themselves or go back to bed – but if a person walks frequently in their sleep they might want to see a doctor, in case they injure themselves falling down the stairs. There is no truth in the myth that waking a sleepwalker is dangerous, but it's often easier to guide them gently back to bed.

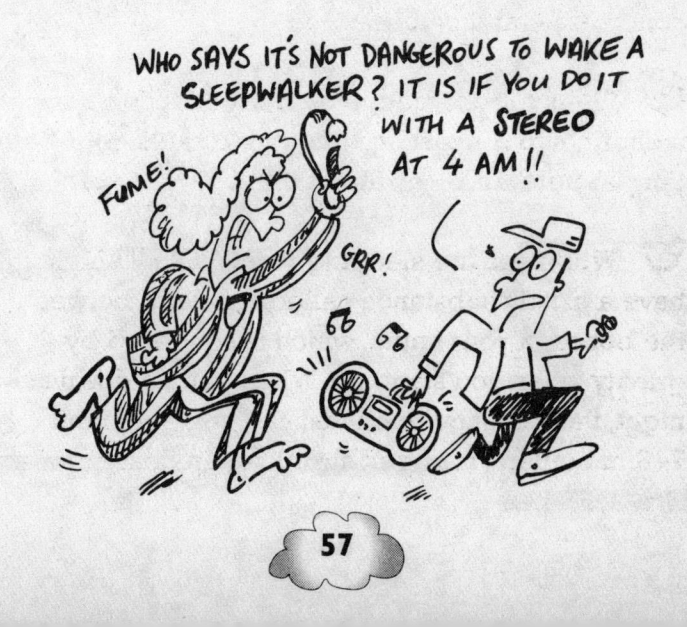

WHO SAYS IT'S NOT DANGEROUS TO WAKE A SLEEPWALKER? IT IS IF YOU DO IT WITH A STEREO AT 4 AM!!

6 While you are sleeping your 'body clock' is ticking away inside your brain. This clock tells your body when to sleep and when to wake up. Unfortunately, it can't tell when you have travelled to a different part of the world, so it can make you want to go to sleep even if it is midday where you are. This feeling is what we call 'jet lag'.

7 We need less and less sleep as we get older. Babies need about 18 hours every day, while for most nine to ten year olds, nine to ten hours of sleep is about right. Adults can manage on eight hours while very old people can make do with about five. When Margaret Thatcher was Prime Minister of Britain she usually slept for only four hours a night. Mind you, with all the things our bodies get up to while we're sleeping, perhaps it's best to wake up so we can get some rest!

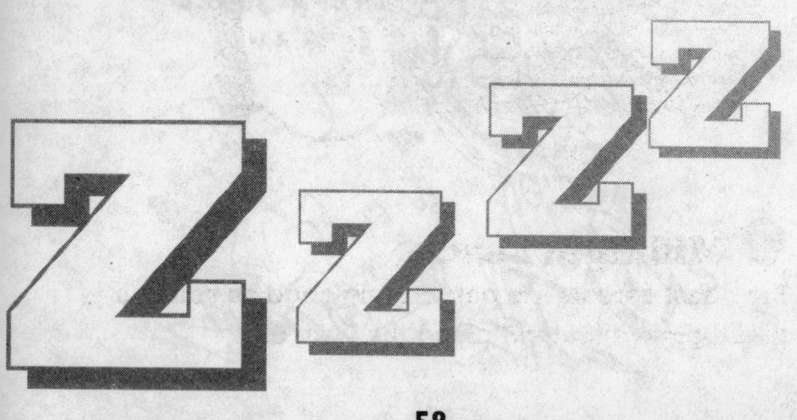

DREAM ON

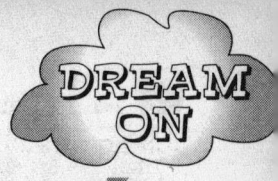

DOZE WERE THE DAYS

Can't get to sleep? Mr Funny's got some tried and tested solutions. You'll soon find that you're...Hey! Wake up when we're talking to you!

❶ Watch TV
Watching TV in bed guarantees you lots of company as no one else in the house will be able to get to sleep either.

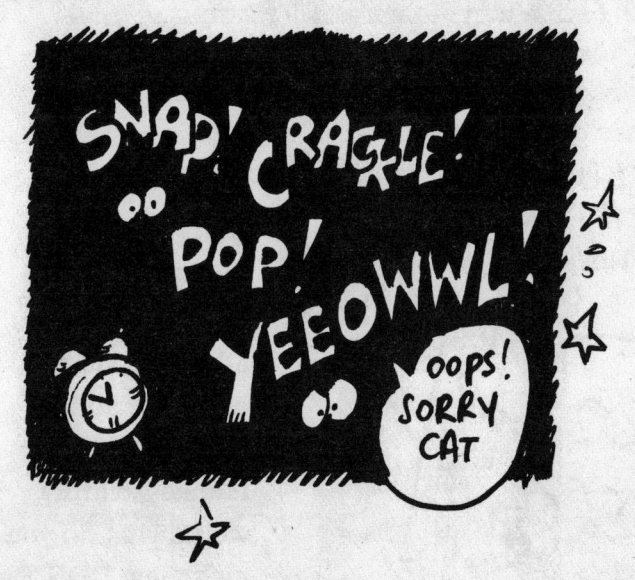

SNAP! CRACKLE! POP! YEEOWWL!

OOPS! SORRY CAT

❷ Midnight snack
Breakfast cereals are particularly good as you can find them without switching the light on.

❸ Count sheep

You'll be so exhausted from carrying all those sheep into your bedroom you'll probably fall asleep anyway.

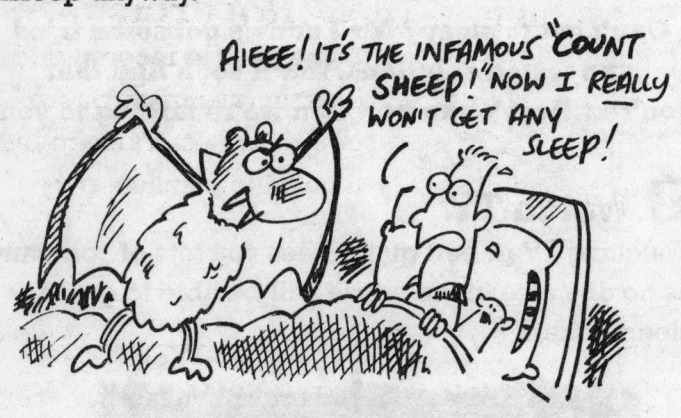

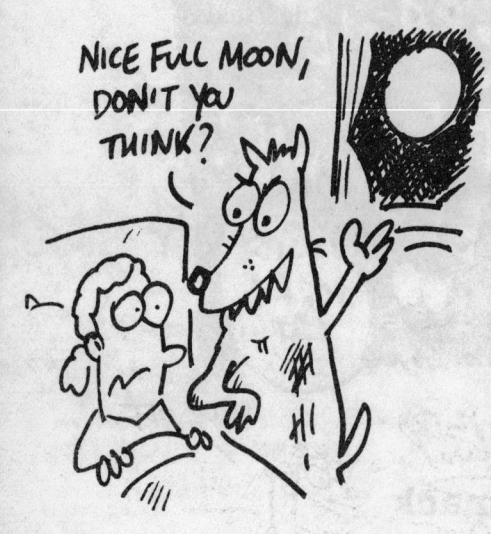

AIEEE! IT'S THE INFAMOUS "COUNT SHEEP"! NOW I REALLY WON'T GET ANY SLEEP!

NICE FULL MOON, DON'T YOU THINK?

❹ Talk to your cuddly toys

Don't be shy – we all like to snuggle up to our cuddly teddy, cuddly monkey, cuddly wolf...what do you mean you DON'T have a cuddly wolf? UH OH!

❺ Read school books

You'll definitely fall asleep...

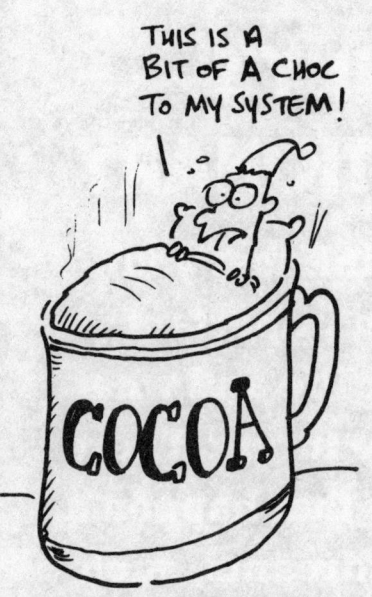

THIS IS A BIT OF A CHOC TO MY SYSTEM!

❻ Hot drinks

Some people recommend a warm mug of cocoa for people who can't sleep but it gets the blankets very soggy.

❼ Self-hypnosis

Only problem is when the alarm goes off, you think you're Elvis Presley.

❽ Rock yourself to sleep

Very popular if you live in an area that's prone to earthquakes.

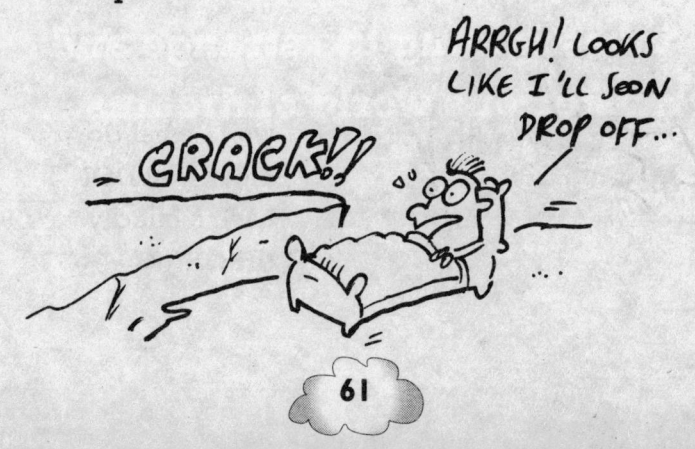

ARRGH! LOOKS LIKE I'LL SOON DROP OFF...

CRACK!!

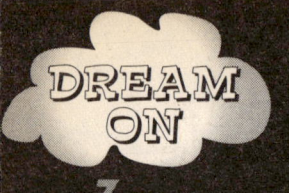

MR FUNNY'S DREAM DICTIONARY

DREAM ON

Many people think that your dreams tell you important things about your life and what may happen in the future. There are certain things that happen a lot in everyone's dreams, such as falling from a cliff or being chased. But what do they actually mean? Mr Funny's been investigating the strange and mysterious world of dreams…

ACCIDENT Dreaming about having an accident doesn't necessarily mean you're going to have one. It may mean that you're going to lose something or that you should be careful about lending money. For instance, if you lend your money to the school bully, you may well have an 'accident' when you try to get it back!

AEROPLANE A dream about an aeroplane is supposed to foretell an exciting adventure. Especially if you wake up in the middle of it and realise that you're supposed to be piloting the plane...

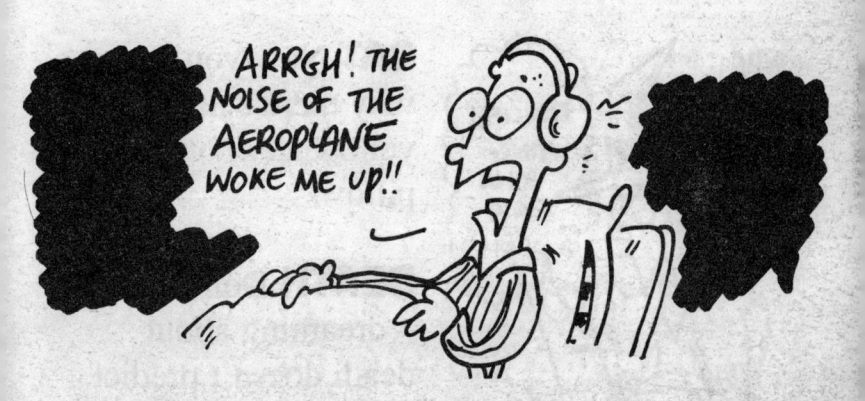

ANGEL Either you are about to fall in love or you've fallen asleep on top of a Christmas tree.

BABY This dream means good luck (either that or your little brother has crawled into your bed again).

BELL Wake up! You're late for school!

BLOOD A little blood in a dream predicts good luck – especially if your name is Dracula.

BOOK This dream means nothing unless of course the book is *The Seriously Funny Guide to Your Body* in which case you should rush out immediately and buy lots more copies.

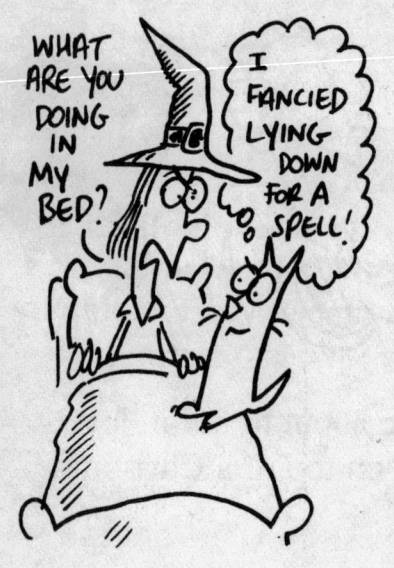

CAT Now you know why there's a funny yellow stain on your pillow.

DEATH Don't panic – dreaming about death doesn't predict death in real life. Instead, it may mean that some kind of change may be necessary. How long have you been wearing that pair of socks?

ELEPHANT Means something important – but we've forgotten what it is.

FALLING Either you're about to have an adventure or you shouldn't lie so close to the edge of your bed.

GHOST Don't watch *The X Files* before going to bed.

NUMBERS If you dream of numbers, it's worth writing them down when you wake up to see if any of them have some special significance in real life. However, if you rush out and spend all your money on lottery tickets, this dream could mean you're going to be broke for quite some time to come.

PAPER If it's blank, you may have fallen asleep while doing your homework. If it says 'School Report' followed by the letter 'F', you definitely did!

QUARREL As dreams usually mean the opposite of what happens in real life, dreaming of a quarrel actually means peace. Yes it does. What do you mean you don't agree? Look, if you're going to argue about it...

ROCK You fell asleep listening to heavy metal on your personal stereo.

SHEEP You can stop counting now, you're asleep.

TEETH To dream about teeth is a good omen. Unless that person called Dracula has woken up from their dream about blood and they're now feeling a bit peckish.

WATER Your hot water bottle's burst.

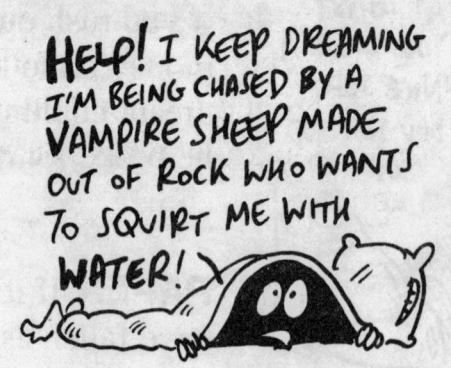

HELP! I KEEP DREAMING I'M BEING CHASED BY A VAMPIRE SHEEP MADE OUT OF ROCK WHO WANTS TO SQUIRT ME WITH WATER!

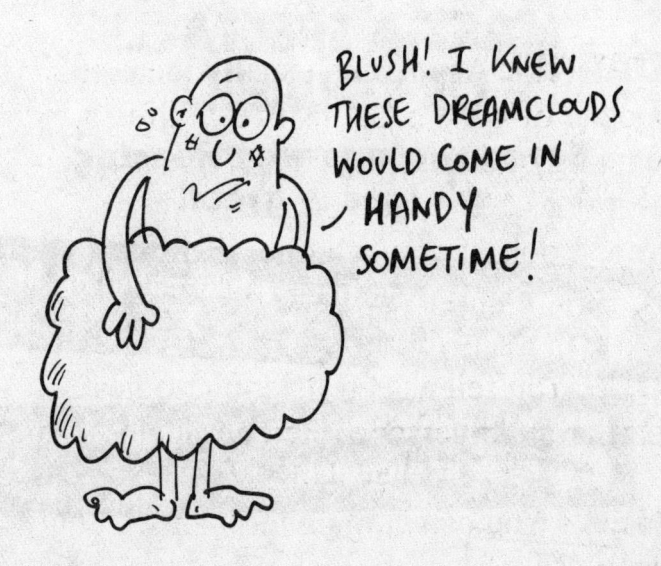

Note: Most of us dream about being caught in the street naked at some time or another. It's a common dream, suggesting that something is worrying us. Don't panic, just pinch yourself and you'll soon wake up. What's that you say? You have pinched yourself and it's not a dream? Well, at least now you know what you've got to worry about!

FACE UP TO IT

MAKE A SPECTACLE OF YOURSELF

Seven reasons why wearing glasses is great!

1 You can start fires while camping in the woods.

2 You don't get bugs flying into your eyes in summer.

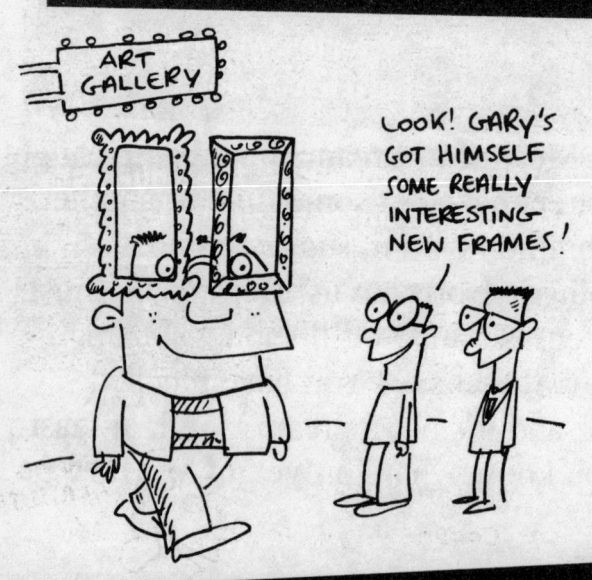

> LOOK! GARY'S GOT HIMSELF SOME REALLY INTERESTING NEW FRAMES!

3 You can do impressions of famous people.

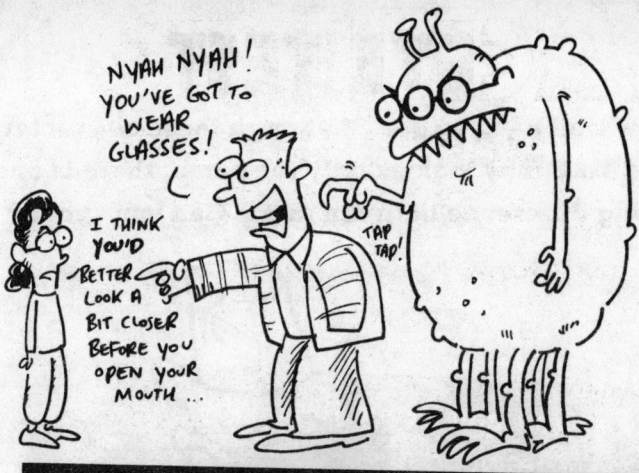

4 You've got an excuse for not doing your homework. (Lost glasses!)

5 You can lend them to your fave star to disguise themselves when they're trying to escape from a mob.

6 You can really look like your pets. (Make them wear glasses too!)

7 You're used to wearing them by the time everyone else has to!

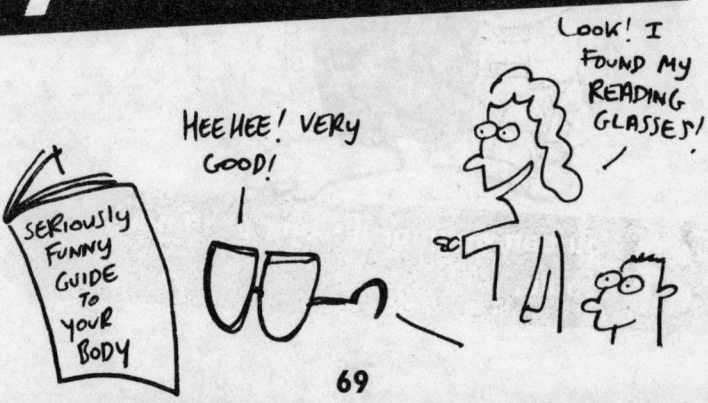

EYE TEST

How well can you see? Although these two pictures of Mr Funny look exactly the same, there is one big difference between them. Can you spot it?

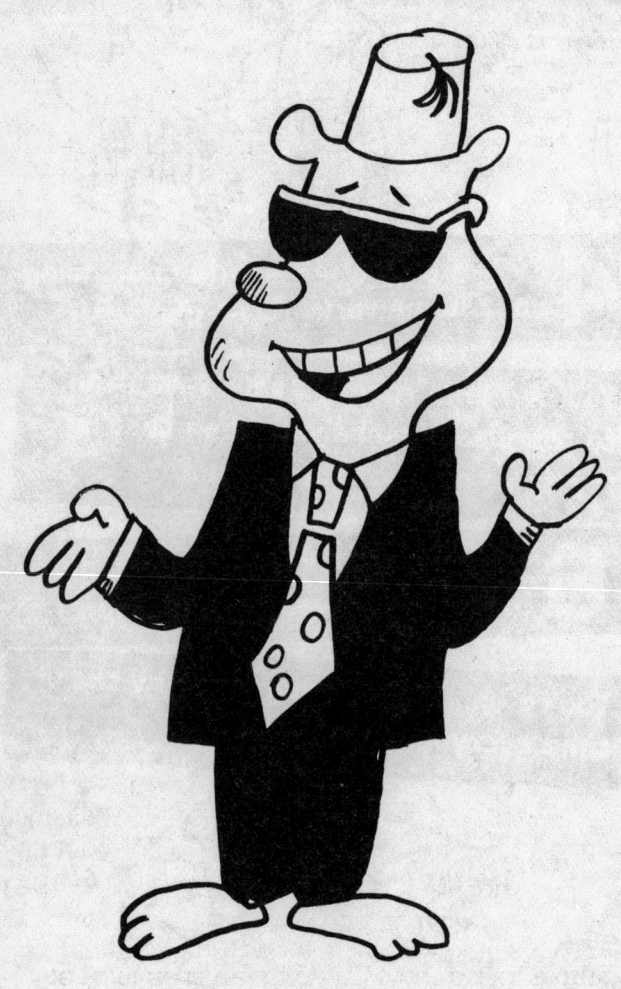

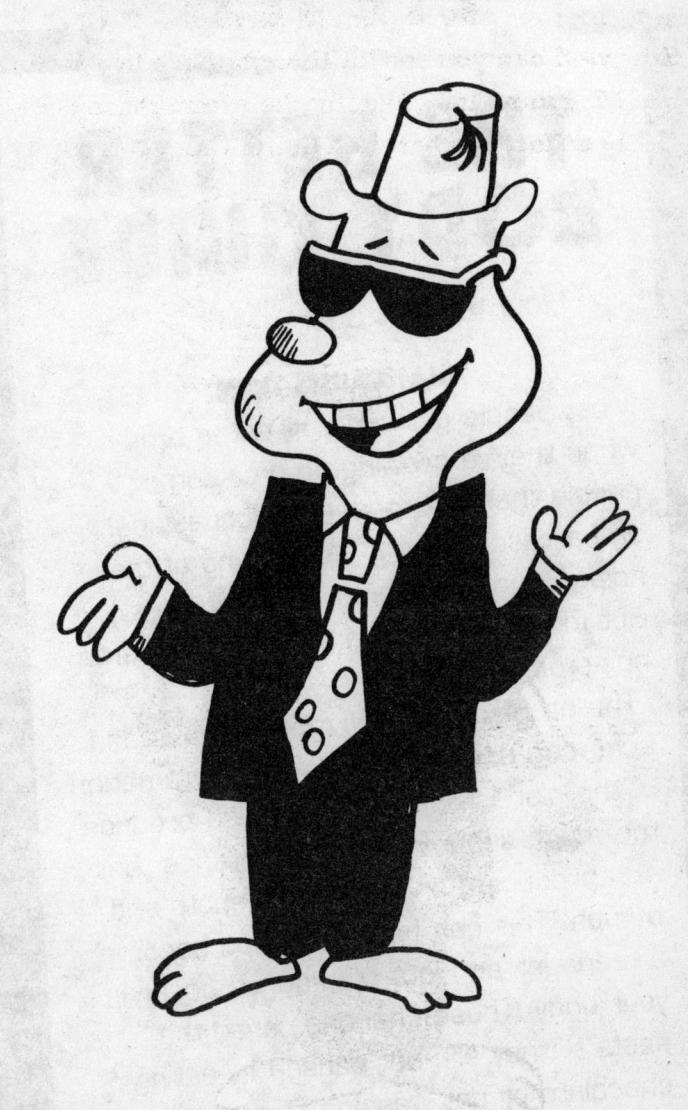

Answer: In the picture on the left page Mr Funny is wearing blue Y-fronts under his suit, but in the picture on the right he is wearing his yellow boxer shorts.

THE BETTER BODY GUIDE

How to sort out SPOTS

WHAT CAUSES THEM?

Most people get spots at some time when they're growing up. For some people that just means the occasional embarrassing bump on the end of the nose (usually just before the big party). But for others, life can suddenly become non-stop spotty hell.

The problem can get more serious and acne can develop. This is an inflammation of the glands on the face, which produce too much sebum (an oily substance that skin produces) and results in spots and bumps. This can happen as you become a teenager and lots of changes occur in your body. These changes cause the spots – they are not caused by eating chocolate or not washing enough. However, a healthy diet and a regular skincare routine is still a good idea and will certainly help fight the spot war.

WHAT TO DO

The good news is there's a lot you can do to get rid of spots and acne. The first thing to remember is DO NOT squeeze or pick your spots. You'll just encourage the spot to spread and become infected. Instead, try some of the many skin care products on the market that contain special anti-spot ingredients such as Benzoyl peroxide and Salicylic acid. These products often come in different strengths, so start off with the weakest and follow the instructions carefully. Don't expect instant results, but persevere and your skin should gradually improve over time.

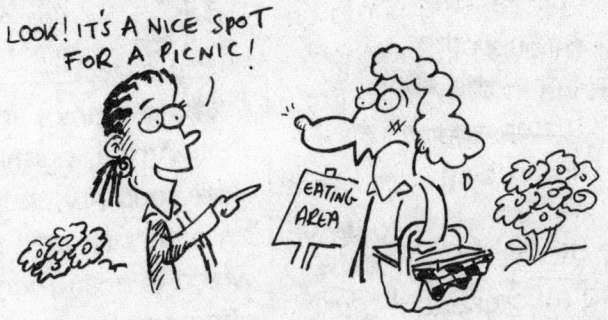

If you think you are suffering from acne or you can't see any improvement in your skin, visit your doctor. There are various treatments which your doctor can prescribe, including antibiotic tablets. Remember, there's no need to suffer in silence!

It is also a good idea to drink lots of water and avoid fatty or fried food. (Good advice for everyone!) Spots can also be made worse by stress, so stop worrying and concentrate on trying out this advice. You'll soon be able to spot the difference.

FUN FACTS

MAKING FACES

❗ Although Beethoven was deaf, he used to put a stick on top of his piano and bite into it. Then he could 'hear' the music through the vibrations in the stick.

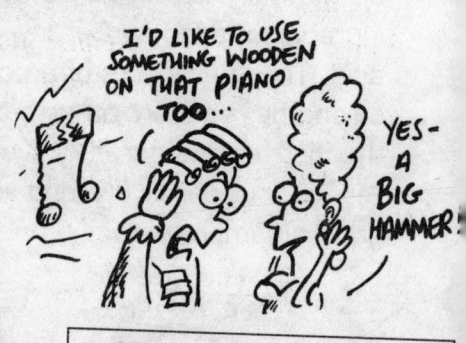

I'D LIKE TO USE SOMETHING WOODEN ON THAT PIANO TOO...

YES — A BIG HAMMER!

❗ In many parts of Africa, people clean their teeth by chewing on a certain kind of stick which is even more effective than a toothbrush.

SOMEONE KEEPS SQUEEZING THE STICK IN THE MIDDLE!

❗ Our nose can distinguish between more than 10,000 different smells.

SMELLS LIKE.... EEK! MY OWN FEET!!

74

- Colour blindness (when you can't tell the difference between certain colours, usually red and green) is ten times more common in boys than in girls.

- Although the rest of our body increases over 20 times in size after we are born, our eyes only increase three and a quarter times in size.

EVER SINCE I FOUND OUT I WAS COLOUR BLIND, I'VE BEEN REALLY BLUE... I MEAN GREEN... OR SHOULD THAT BE RED?

- In some parts of Japan, it used to be fashionable for girls to tattoo a moustache on their upper lip.

- In ninth century Ireland, the Vikings imposed a 'nose tax'. If you couldn't pay it, you had your nose cut off!

ALL I SAID WAS "THOSE VIKINGS REALLY GET UP MY NOSE!"

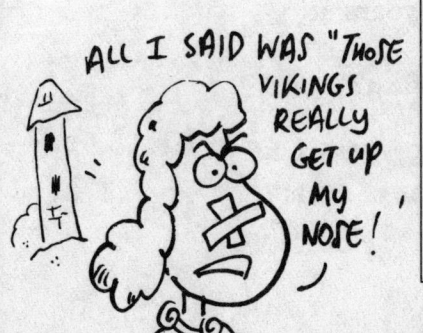

- Queen Elizabeth I used to stuff her mouth with cloth to disguise the fact that she had no front teeth, while George Washington's false teeth were made of wood.

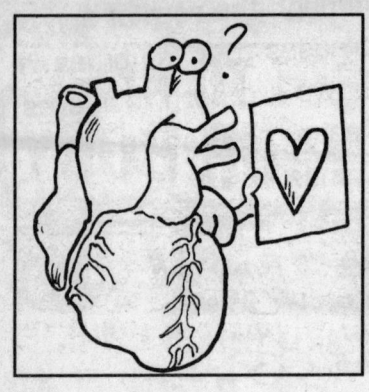

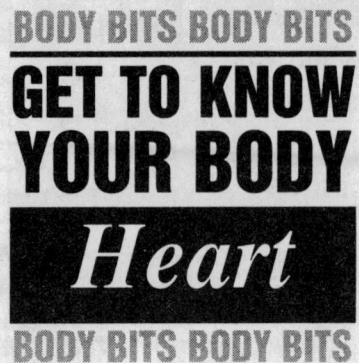

BODY BITS BODY BITS
GET TO KNOW YOUR BODY
Heart
BODY BITS BODY BITS

Name: Heart
What's your favourite food?
Beat Root, Heart-ichokes, Pump-kin.
What's your best quality?
You can't live without me.
What's your worst habit?
I'm sometimes very quick to attack.
Do you like travelling?
Yes, as long as it's by Blood Vessel.
Favourite sports?
Quiet ones - I'm easily broken.
What annoys you?
People who wear me on their sleeve –
it's freezing in winter!
What's your favourite hobby?
Painting – I've spent a few years at
heart college.
What's your favourite saying?
'Beats me!'

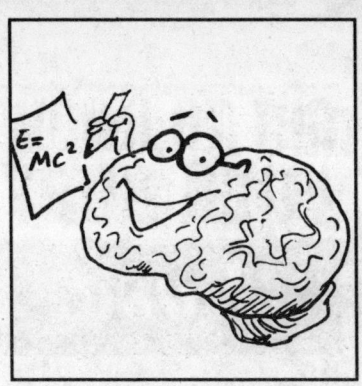

BODY BITS BODY BITS
GET TO KNOW YOUR BODY
Brain
BODY BITS BODY BITS

Name: Brain
What's your favourite hobby?
I'm thinking, I'm thinking...hang on, that is my hobby!
What's your favourite song?
Braindrops Are Falling On My Head.
What's your favourite food?
(Head)bangers and mash.
What's your favourite sport?
Surfing, especially on brainwaves.
What's your best quality?
I'm a quick thinker.
What's your worst quality?
I can sometimes be a headache.
What annoys you?
Brain teasers – I hate it when they shout, 'Brains are grey and lumpy, nyah, nyah, nyah!'
Do you think you'll ever be famous?
No, most people like to keep me under their hat.
What's your favourite saying?
'I think I'm going out of my head.'

BODY BITS BODY BITS
GET TO KNOW YOUR BODY
Nose
BODY BITS BODY BITS

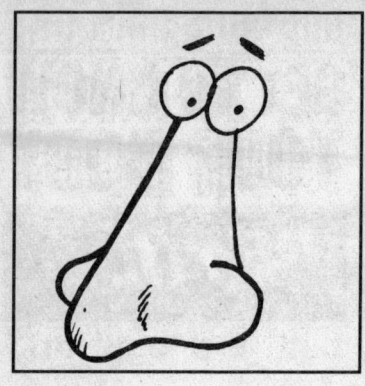

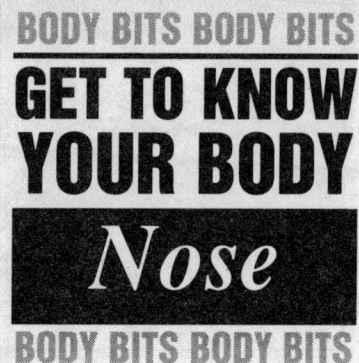

Name: Nose
What's your favourite food?
Breath and butter.
What's your favourite song?
For Sneeze a Jolly Good Fellow.
What's your favourite hobby?
Travelling – you could say I'm a roamin' nose.
What's your favourite movie?
Saturday Night Hayfever.
Who's your favourite movie star?
Sneezy from *Snow White and the Seven Dwarfs*.
He just blows me away.
What's your best quality?
I can sniff out a bargain.
What's your worst quality?
I sometimes poke myself into other people's business.
What are your predictions for the future?
What would I know about the future?
I'm not Nostril-damus!
What's your favourite saying?
'Atishoo!'

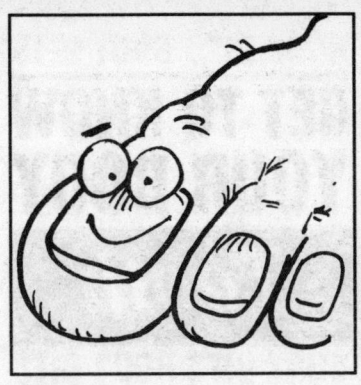

GET TO KNOW YOUR BODY
Big Toe

Name: Big Toe
What's your favourite food?
Toe-mato ketchup.
What's your favourite sport?
Football. (I always get a kick out of it.)
What's your favourite hobby?
Collecting stamps.
What's your favourite music?
Sole music.
What's your best quality?
I stick out from the rest.
What's your worst habit?
I sometimes get too big for my boots.
Is your job hard?
Believe me you wouldn't want to be in my shoes.
How did you build up your career?
Step by step.
Where do you drink?
Heel bars.
What annoys you most?
Ankles – they're always following me around.
What's your favourite saying?
'Toe be or not toe be...'

BODY BITS BODY BITS
GET TO KNOW YOUR BODY
Tooth
BODY BITS BODY BITS

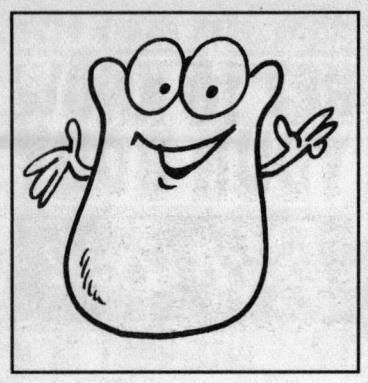

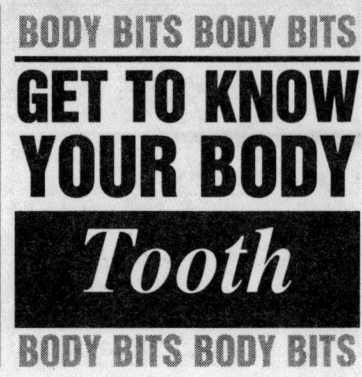

Name: Tooth
What's your favourite food?
Gum.
What's your favourite hobby?
Computer games (I love those bytes!).
What's your favourite song?
Blue Suede Chews.
What's your best quality?
I'm very sweet.
What's your worst habit?
I'm always down in the mouth
What annoys you most?
Other teeth – they can be very false.
Do you think you will ever be famous?
I'm already at the tip of everyone's tongue.
What do you think of dentists' drills?
Boring.
So you don't enjoy going to the dentist then?
No, it leaves me numb.
What's your favourite saying?
'The Molar the Merrier.'

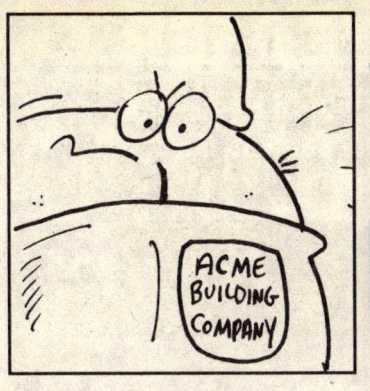

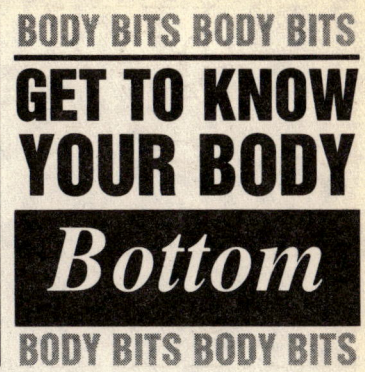

BODY BITS BODY BITS
GET TO KNOW YOUR BODY
Bottom
BODY BITS BODY BITS

Name: Bottom
What's your favourite food?
Hot Cross Bums.
What's your favourite hobby?
Sitting in front of the TV – or sitting anywhere else for that matter.
What's your best quality?
Whatever you do, I'll be right behind you.
What's your worst habit?
I can be a bit of a stinker.
What annoys you most?
The nose, eyes and ears – they're always looking down on me.
How do you react?
I turn the other cheek.
Do you regret this later on?
Yes – in fact I could kick myself.
What are your favourite fashions?
I always look good in trousers.
What's your favourite line from a song?
'And now the end is near...'

BRAINTEASER

Mr Funny has drawn some mind-boggling bones.
Can you spot the odd one out?

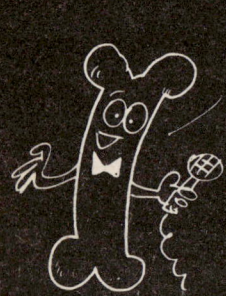

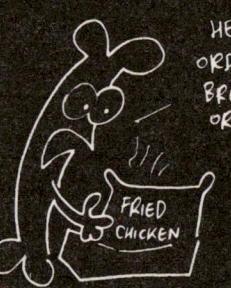

HEY! I DIDN'T ORDER ANY BREASTS, WINGS OR DRUMSTICKS!

FRIED CHICKEN

HAVE YOU HEARD THE ONE ABOUT THE BLOCKED NOSE? IT'LL TAKE YOUR BREATH AWAY?

2. Thigh bone

1. Funny bone

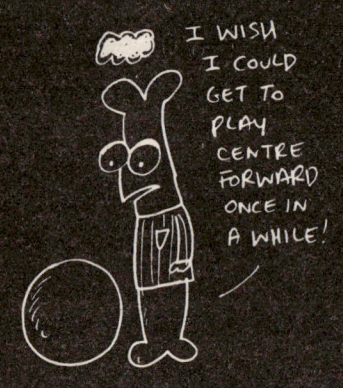

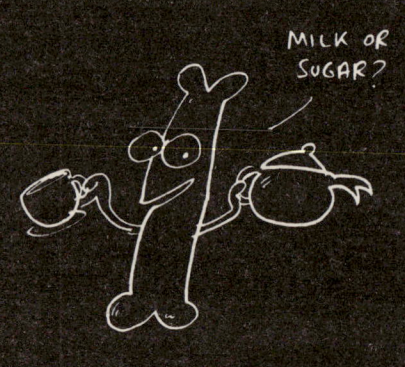

MILK OR SUGAR?

I WISH I COULD GET TO PLAY CENTRE FORWARD ONCE IN A WHILE!

4. T-bone

3. Back bone

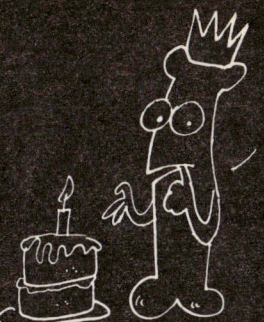

5. Hip bone

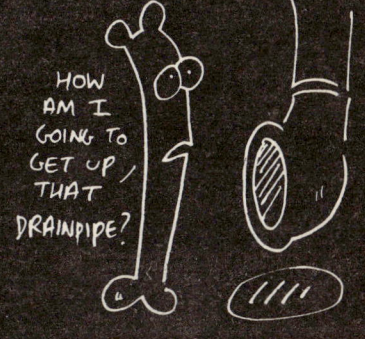

6. Shin bone

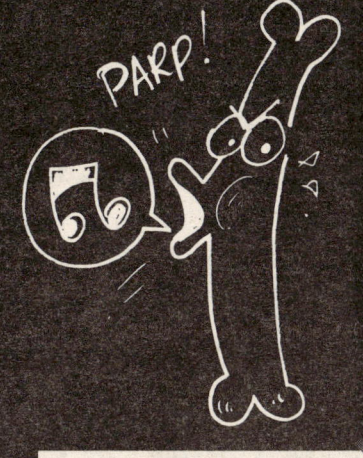

7. Trom-bone

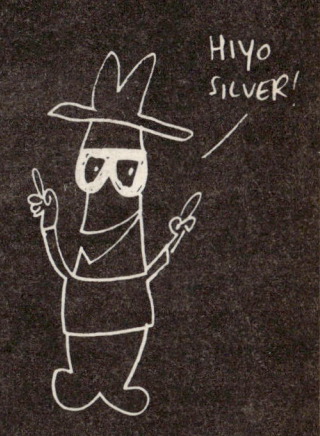

7. The Bone Ranger

Answer: No 6. Mr Funny drew this one on Monday. All the other ones were drawn on Tuesday morning.

YOUNG AND OLD
YOU'VE COME A LONG WAY BABY

You do the most growing and developing you'll ever do in the first ten years of your life. Let's celebrate your achievements.

❶ When you were a baby you couldn't walk on your own.
Now you can. (Unless you've got roller blades.)

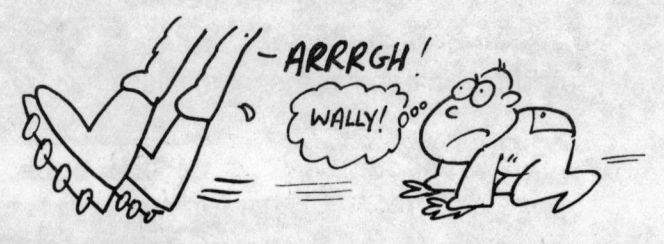

❷ When you were a baby your mum and dad couldn't understand you.
Now they can. (Well, some of the time.)

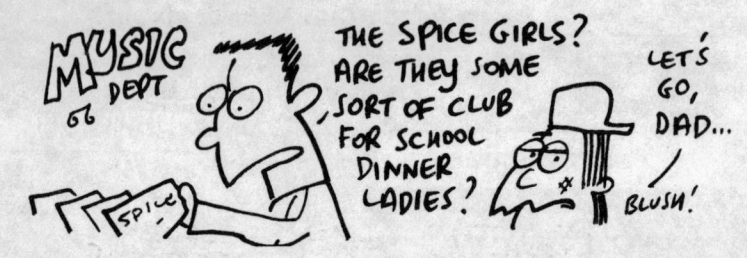

❸ When you were a baby you liked to play with toys.
Now you don't, unless it's the latest 75 byte Mega Shoot-Em-Up platform game.

❹ When you were a baby you cried a lot.
Now you don't, unless one of the soaps is on.

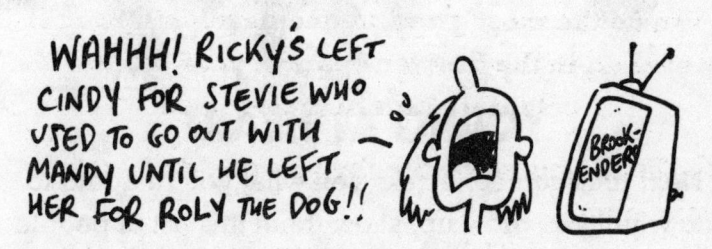

WAHHH! Ricky's left Cindy for Stevie who used to go out with Mandy until he left her for Roly the dog!!

Brook-Enders

❺ When you were a baby you had to be carried around all the time.
Now you don't, unless it's a school morning.

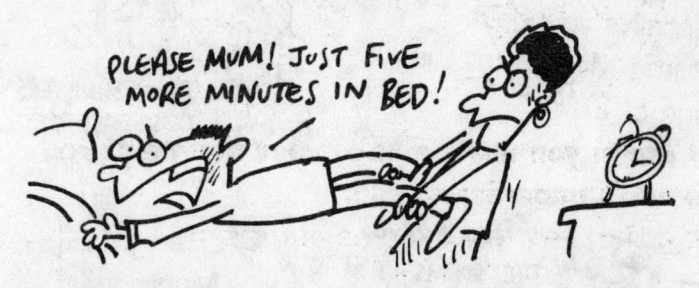

PLEASE MUM! JUST FIVE MORE MINUTES IN BED!

❻ When you were a baby you liked playing with cuddly toys.
Now you still like cuddly toys – and it's the same old whiffy one, too.

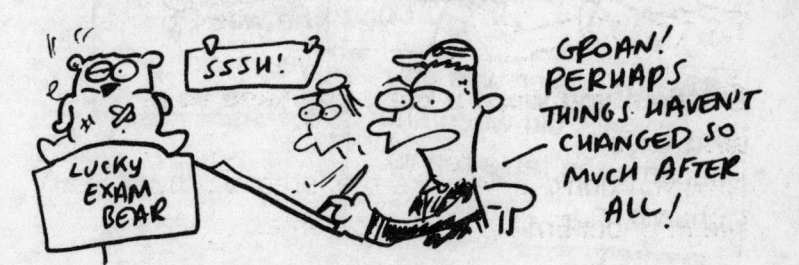

LUCKY EXAM BEAR

SSSH!

GROAN! PERHAPS THINGS HAVEN'T CHANGED SO MUCH AFTER ALL!

FUN FACTS

YOUNG AT HEART

Next time someone asks you what you're going to do when you grow up, show them this list of people who didn't bother to wait around.

> ❗ William Pitt the Younger became Britain's youngest Prime Minister at the age of 24.

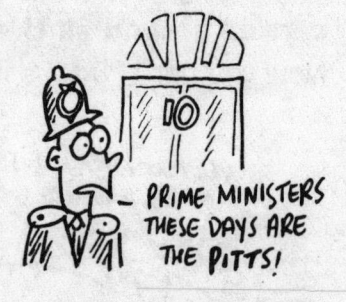

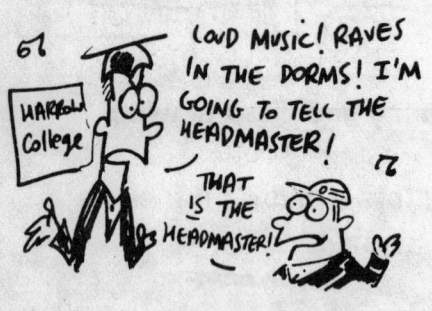

— PRIME MINISTERS THESE DAYS ARE THE PITTS!

LOUD MUSIC! RAVES IN THE DORMS! I'M GOING TO TELL THE HEADMASTER!

THAT IS THE HEADMASTER!

> ❗ Henry Montague was made headmaster of Harrow College when he was 26 years old.

> ❗ Joy Foster was only eight years old when she became the table tennis champion of Jamaica.

❣ Pope Benedict IX took the throne when he was 12 years old – and was later sacked for corruption!

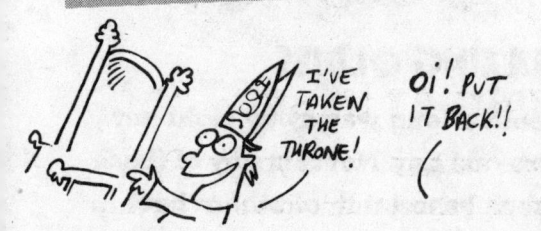

I'VE TAKEN THE THRONE!

OI! PUT IT BACK!!

❣ A woman in Leicester worked for the same elastic company from the time she was nine until she was 95 years old.

❣ Henry III became King of England when he was only ten months old.

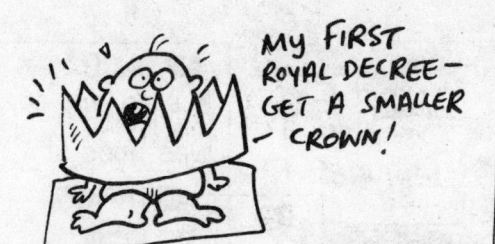

MY FIRST ROYAL DECREE – GET A SMALLER CROWN!

❣ By the he time she was 22, Lucrezia Borgia had been married four times.

❣ The German writer, Goethe, wrote a story in seven different languages when he was only ten years old.

GOETHE! DID YOU WRITE THAT STORY ON MY @#$@ CLEAN WALL?

GOSH! MUM'S USING LANGUAGE EVEN I DON'T KNOW..

FUN FACTS

AMAZING OLDIES

Being old may seem a long way away right now, but you'll get there one day. Not that any of these super senior citizens have let it 'old them back...

> ♥ At 90, Pablo Picasso was still turning out paintings.

> ♥ At 91, Adolph Zukor was boss of Paramount Pictures.

> ♥ Pianist Arthur Rubinstein gave one of his greatest performances at Carnegie Hall aged 89.

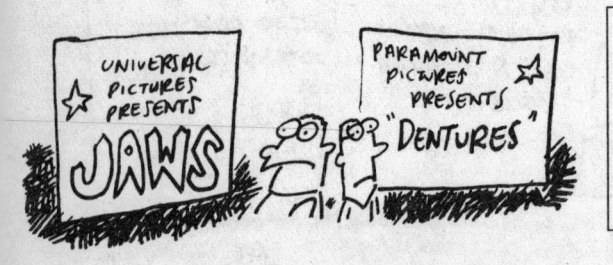

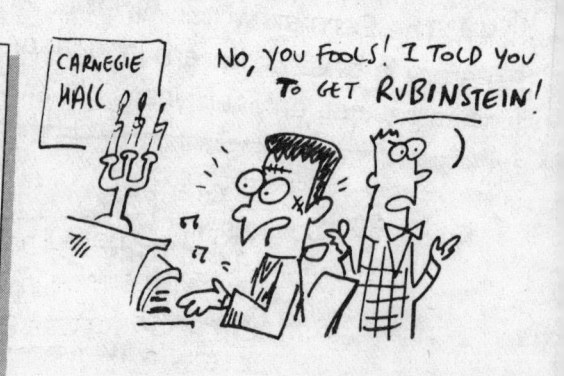

❤ Pepi II was Pharaoh of Egypt from 2278 to 2184 B.C. – an amazing 94 years.

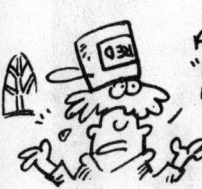

ALL I SAID WAS "MICHELANGELO, I DON'T LIKE THE COLOUR YOU'VE PICKED FOR THE CEILING."

❤ Michelangelo, the Italian sculptor, was still designing churches aged 88.

❤ Coco Chanel (of Chanel perfume fame) was head of her fashion design company at the age of 85.

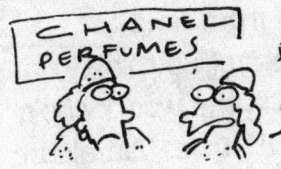

CHANEL PERFUMES

DON'T TELL THE BOSS SHE'S TOO OLD OR SHE'LL REALLY KICK UP A STINK!

❤ At 76, Nelson Mandela became President of South Africa, after spending 27 years in prison for fighting against apartheid.

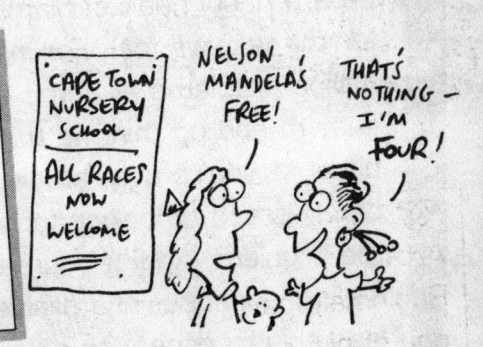

CAPE TOWN NURSERY SCHOOL – ALL RACES NOW WELLCOME

NELSON MANDELA'S FREE!

THAT'S NOTHING – I'M FOUR!

❤ Comedian George Burns won an Oscar for his performance in *The Sunshine Boys* when he was 80.

THE BETTER BODY GUIDE

How to Blast the Blues

WHAT CAUSES THEM

Everybody gets the blues at one time or another, whatever age they are. Growing up can be a difficult time and it's quite normal to feel a bit low from time to time. Unfortunately, most of us think we're the ONLY person in the world who's ever felt down, which isn't true. We also have a nasty habit of blaming ourselves for the way we feel. For instance, if you're having problems at home or at school it's easy to end up thinking the problems are because you're ugly/stupid/just plain bad, instead of looking for ways to solve the problem. And of course, once you're feeling low about one problem you're even less able to cope with other problems and the whole thing becomes a depressing gloomy mess...AAARGH!

WHAT TO DO

The more you concentrate on the bad things in life, the worse you'll feel. In the same way, the more you concentrate on the good stuff, the better you'll feel. Make a list of all the talents you have (and you do have them – you're smart enough to be reading a *Seriously Funny Guide* for a start). Think of all the good points about your personality as well. You may not be brilliant at chemistry but you might well be brilliant at solving your friends' problems and being a good listener.

Being happy depends a lot on how you look at things. For instance, if you're having problems with maths, which of these do you think would be the best way of looking at it?

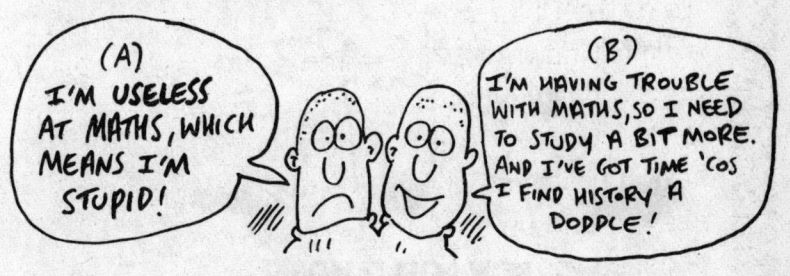

(A) I'M USELESS AT MATHS, WHICH MEANS I'M STUPID!

(B) I'M HAVING TROUBLE WITH MATHS, SO I NEED TO STUDY A BIT MORE. AND I'VE GOT TIME 'COS I FIND HISTORY A DODDLE!

No points for guessing 'B'!

If you have a problem that's really worrying you, do talk to someone about it. If there's no one you can talk to at home, try one of your teachers. You could also phone *Childline* (0800 111111) where someone will listen and try to help you.

Most importantly of all, smile. Remember – not only does it make you feel better, it makes everyone else wonder what you've been up to...

Tricky Tricks **AND** Phenomenal Feats

HOW TO HAVE TWO NOSES

This is a simple trick but it will give you a really weird feeling. Simply cross your fingers, close your eyes and rub your crossed fingers over the tip of your nose as shown. You should find that you can feel two noses. The same applies if you rub your crossed fingers on a snooker or golf ball.

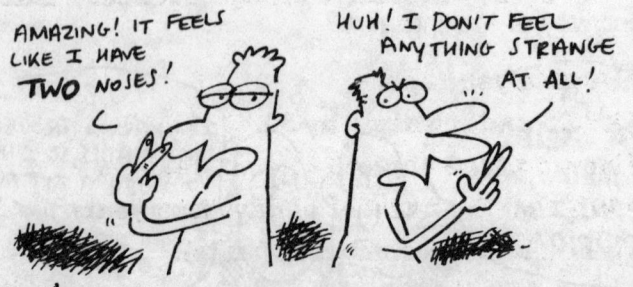

HOW DOES IT WORK?

The touch sensors in your fingertips send messages back to the brain – but of course the sensors don't 'know' that you've crossed your fingers, so they each send a separate message. That's why your brain thinks it can feel two noses.

You could try blindfolding a friend and telling them to cross their fingers, then give them a ball to feel. Do they feel one ball or two? It's easy when you 'nose' how!

OUTR-AGE-OUS!

How long have you been in your body? If you're seven years old, not as long as you think. Every cell in your body replaces itself every seven years, so chances are you're still pretty much a brand new you!

However, you can still use your age and some coins to do this amazing trick. (You may need to use a calculator in case your brain isn't quite as brand new as the rest of you.)

❶ **Take some change out of your pocket or purse – any amount as long as it's less than £1.**
❷ **Double your age.**
❸ **Add 5 and multiply by 50.**
❹ **Now add the amount of your change.**
❺ **Subtract the number of days in a year (not a leap year, smarty pants).**
❻ **Add 115.**
❼ **Divide by 100.**
❽ **Your result will be your age, then a decimal point, then the amount of change you have.**

LET ME KNOW IF THIS WORKS – I HAD TO USE ALL MY CHANGE TO BUY THE CALCULATOR!

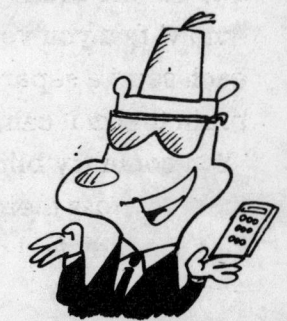

Tricky Tricks AND Phenomenal Feats

I WANT MY MUMMY!

Here's a bit of body magic which has been around for a long time (several thousand years or so) but done properly, it can still raise a shriek.

HOW TO DO IT

Tell your friends that you've got a very sore finger. While they make the proper sympathetic noises, you can add 'I found it on the floor of the British Museum'.

With a flourish, you take a mysterious box out of your pocket and open it to reveal a real human finger. If your friends don't faint at this stage, go on to tell them that it's the finger of Pharaoh Im-Ho-Tep of ancient Egypt and that there's a rumour that some day the Pharaoh is coming back to get it.

Your friends may not believe you, so you can invite the braver ones to touch the finger – and as they do it will begin to MOVE!

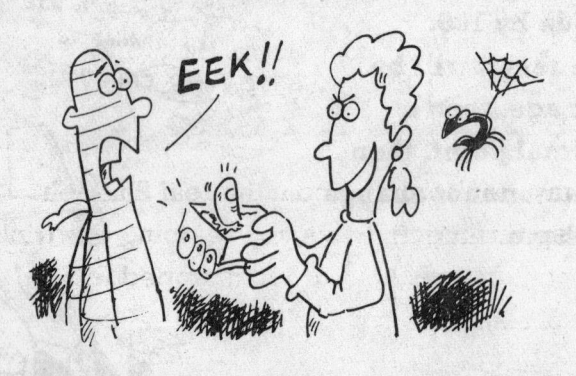

HOW IT'S DONE

Tricky Tricks AND Phenomenal Feats

To pull off this fiendish feat all you need is an ordinary matchbox, your finger and some acting ability.

1. Cut a hole in the bottom of the matchbox as shown (be careful – if you really cut your finger off, there'll be no point doing the trick).

2. Now put your thumb through the hole. Fill the space around the thumb with cotton wool or some other material. You can even dab some tomato ketchup round your knuckle for extra yukky effect. You may also want to paint your fingernail and thumb with make-up or flour to give it that special 'Dead for Several Thousand Years' look.

3. Now decorate the outside of the matchbox with Egyptian symbols or just paint it black. If you hold the whole thing as shown, you will have a very realistic mummy's finger.

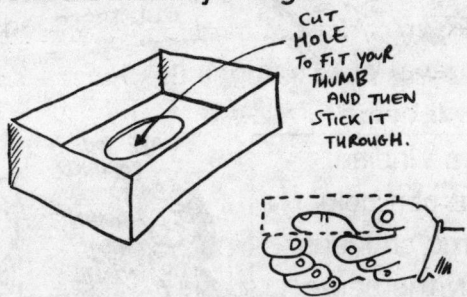

CUT HOLE TO FIT YOUR THUMB AND THEN STICK IT THROUGH.

By the way, don't worry about the real Pharaoh Im-Ho-Tep turning up while you're doing this trick. Like most mummies he's far too wrapped up in himself to bother.

FUN FACTS

BUSY BODIES

Don't try any of these feats at home!

❗ Filipino people in ancient times developed a very fearsome weapon to fight their enemies – today we know it as the yo-yo!

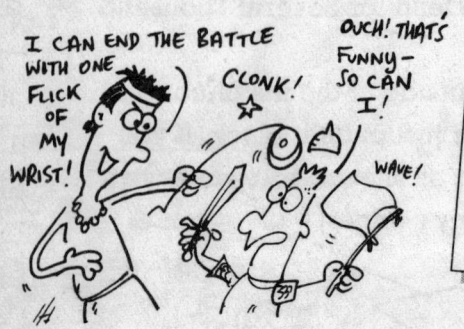

❗ Thomas Topham, an eighteenth-century strongman, could snap his fingers while a man danced on each of his outstretched arms.

❗ Some Indian holy men can hold their arms and legs in exactly the same position for several years.

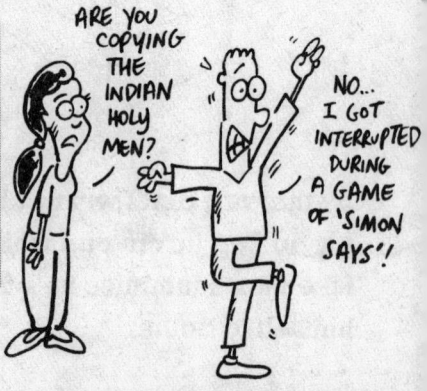

❤ In the early 1900s, there was a 14-year-old French girl who could move heavy furniture using the static electrical current running through her body.

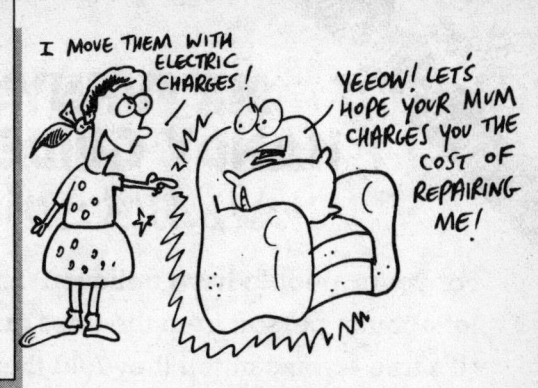

❤ Tennis champion Big Bill Tilden could hit a ball at 214 km per hour.

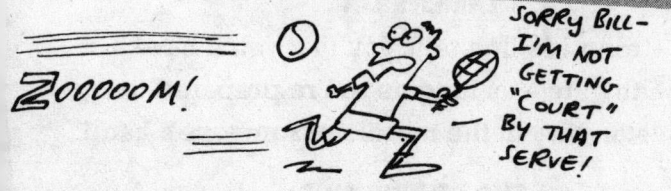

❤ Charles Blondin, a famous acrobat in the nineteenth century, could turn a back somersault while he was on stilts.

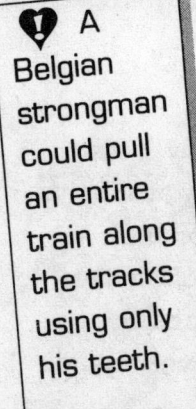

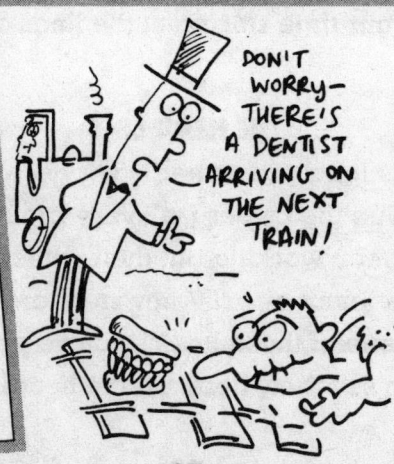

❤ A Belgian strongman could pull an entire train along the tracks using only his teeth.

❤ An Austrian man once walked on his hands for 55 days.

Tricky Tricks AND Phenomenal Feats

MR FUNNY'S HANDY GUIDE TO PALMREADING

For years, people have believed that you can tell a lot about a person from the lines on their hand. (It's true – you can tell they fold their hands a lot.) Examine your right hand and check it against our handy guide below.

THE LIFE LINE

A long, strong life line tells you that you'll have a long healthy life – as long as you're prepared to spend it standing in the middle of someone's hand.

THE DESTINY LINE

This tells you whether or not your life will be calm and peaceful. (Although we can't predict many exciting things happening to you if you're going to spend all your time staring at the lines on your hand.)

THE HEAD LINE

If this line is long, the owner is very brainy. If it's long and blue the owner isn't very brainy as they've obviously been working out their sums on their hand with a leaky biro. TV newsreaders often have more than one of these lines – you've probably heard them say 'Now here are the headlines again'.

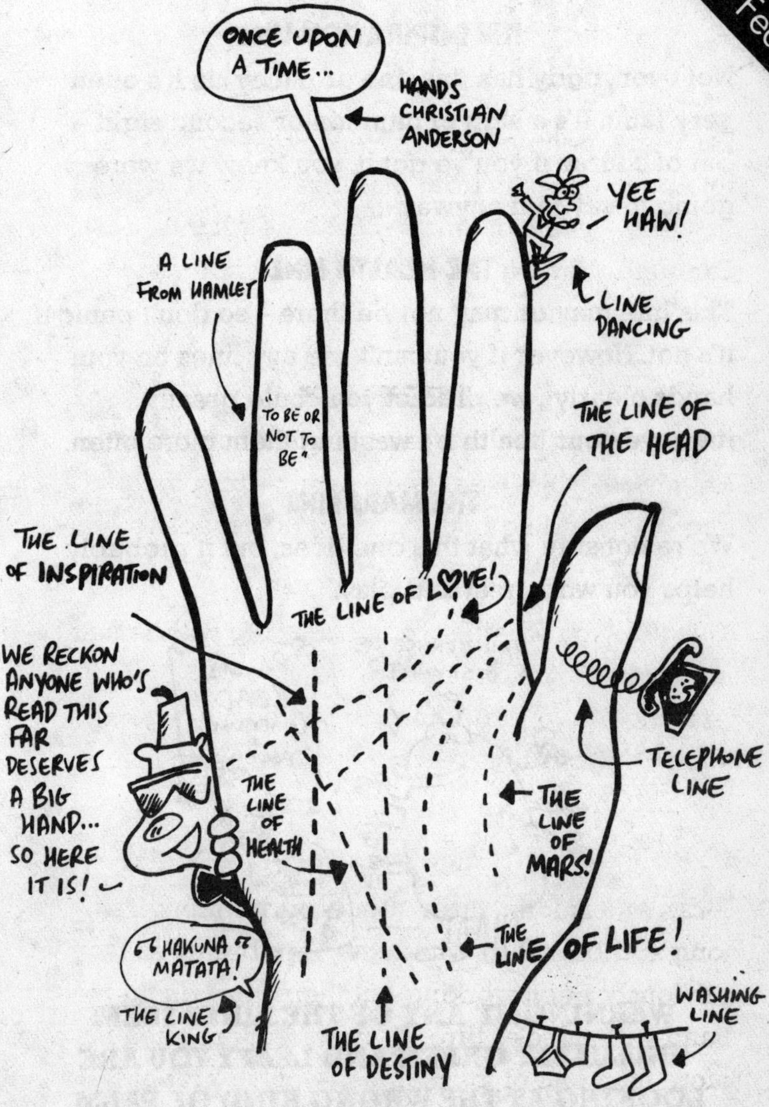
ONCE UPON A TIME...
HANDS CHRISTIAN ANDERSON
YEE HAW!
LINE DANCING
A LINE FROM HAMLET
"TO BE OR NOT TO BE"
THE LINE OF THE HEAD
THE LINE OF INSPIRATION
THE LINE OF LOVE!
WE RECKON ANYONE WHO'S READ THIS FAR DESERVES A BIG HAND... SO HERE IT IS!
TELEPHONE LINE
THE LINE OF HEALTH
THE LINE OF MARS!
HAKUNA MATATA!
THE LINE OF LIFE!
THE LINE KING
WASHING LINE
THE LINE OF DESTINY

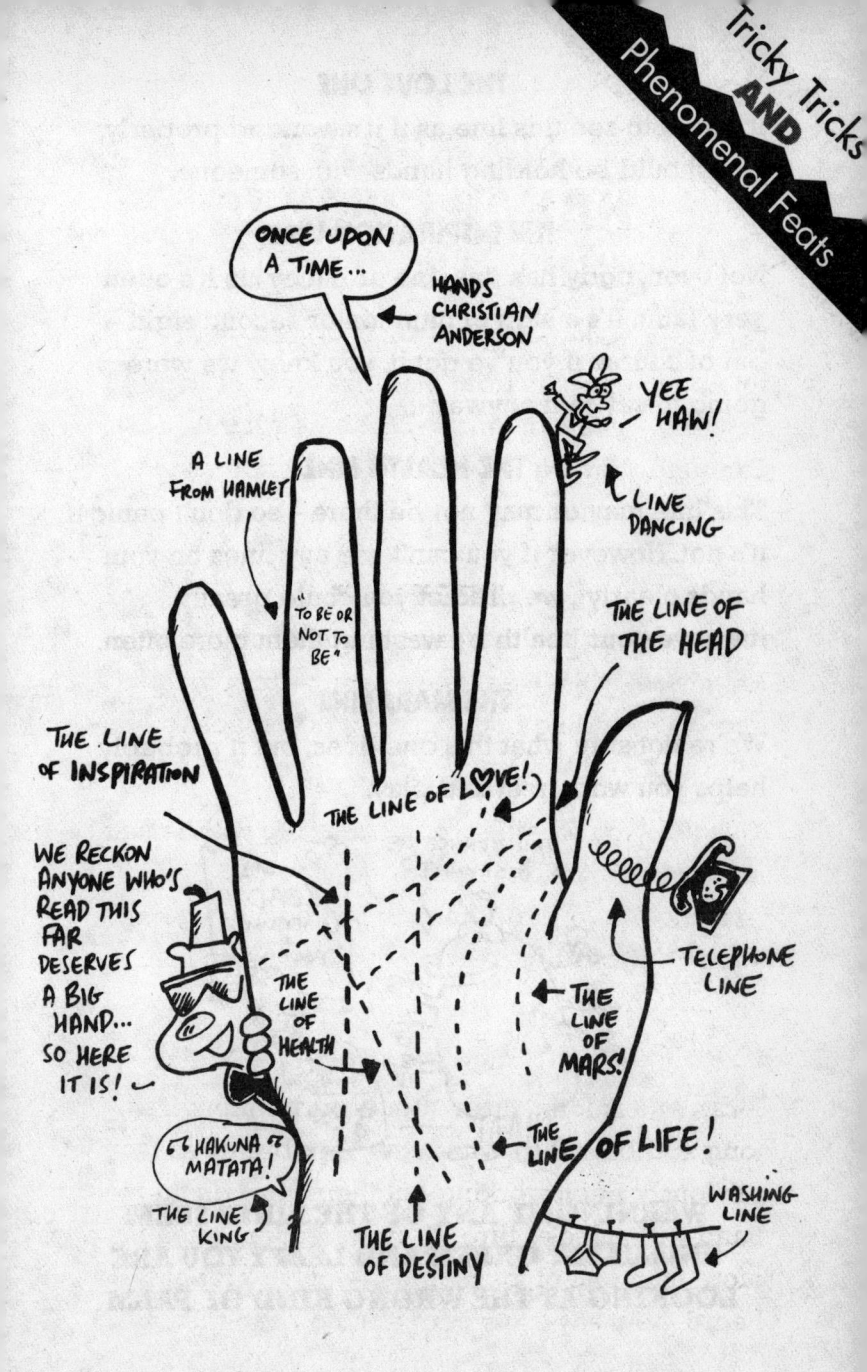

THE LOVE LINE

It's hard to see this line as if it's working properly, you should be holding hands with someone.

THE INSPIRATION LINE

Not everybody has this line or if they do it's often very faint. It's a sign of intuition or second sight – but of course if you've got it, you knew we were going to say that anyway...

THE HEALTH LINE

This line may or may not be there – so don't panic if it's not. However if you can't see any lines on your hands clearly , we predict you could greatly improve your health by washing them more often.

THE MARS LINE

We're not sure what this one does, but it probably helps you work, rest and play.

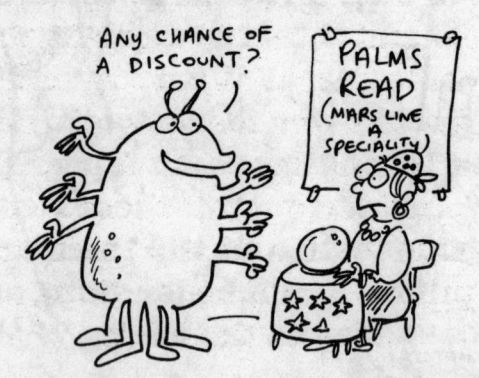

WARNING: IF ANY OF THE LINES SEEM UNUSUALLY GREEN AND LEAFY YOU ARE LOOKING AT THE WRONG KIND OF PALM.

MIGHTY MOLARS

VERY UNFAIR-Y

Have you ever left your tooth under the pillow and received a bright shiny 50- pence piece? What a swizz, eh? Next time you lose a tooth, don't bother letting the tooth fairy rip you off. Instead cut out these really valuable teeth and slip them under your pillow. You'll be laughing all the way to the bank.

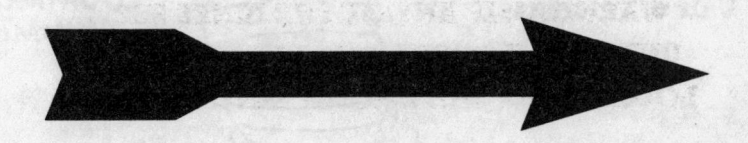

MOVIE 'STUNT' TOOTH
You often see this flying out of someone's mouth when Arnold Schwarzenegger punches them.
Salary: £3,000,000 per picture.

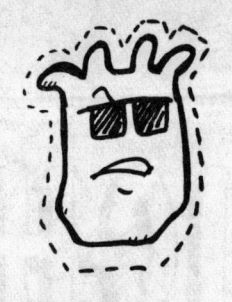

I'LL BE BACK (FOR A CHECK UP IN SIX MONTHS!)

WATCH IT, FAIRY

IF I BITE YOU, YOU'LL BE DINO-SORE!

JURASSIC TOOTH
65 million years old (found embedded in a 65-million-year-old caveman). **Value:** £65,000,000 a piece. **(only £1 per year – what a bargain!)**

TOOTH-ANKHAMUN
Comes ready-wrapped.
Value: Priceless.

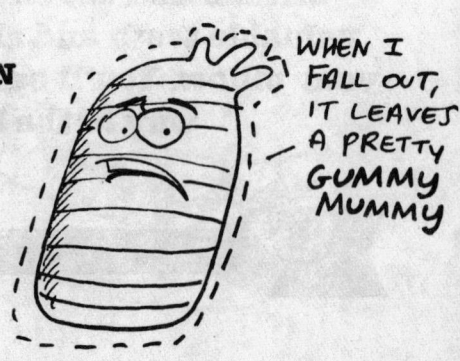

WHEN I FALL OUT, IT LEAVES A PRETTY GUMMY MUMMY

THE TOOTH, THE WHOLE TOOTH AND NOTHING BUT THE TOOTH
Famous for appearing in court (and also bad jokes).
Legal fees: £40,000.

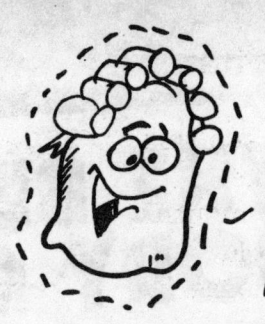

ORDER IN COURT! (MIND YOU, I WOULDN'T HAVE COME OUT IF YOU HADN'T ORDERED SO MUCH STICKY CAKE!

CANINE TOOTH
(Okay, it's not actually worth anything, but if you don't pay up, fairy, I'll get my canine to bite you!)

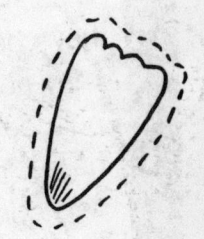

HOPE THAT TOOTH FAIRY SHOWS UP SOON — I FANCY SOME ELF FOOD!

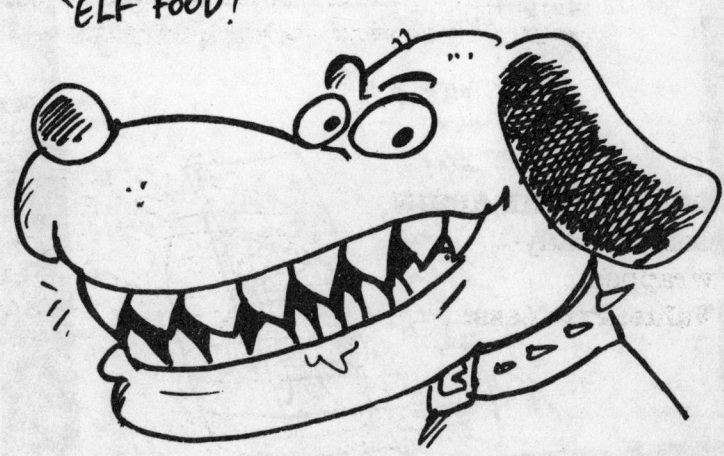

THE BETTER BODY GUIDE

How to beat BAD BREATH

WHAT CAUSES IT?

It can be a bit hard to work out if you have bad breath as even your best friends may not want to tell you. But if you've noticed that people seem a bit reluctant to have close conversations with you, perhaps you should try this test yourself. Cup your hands around your nose and mouth, breathe out and then sniff – if your reaction is 'URRRGH!', perhaps you need to do something about it.

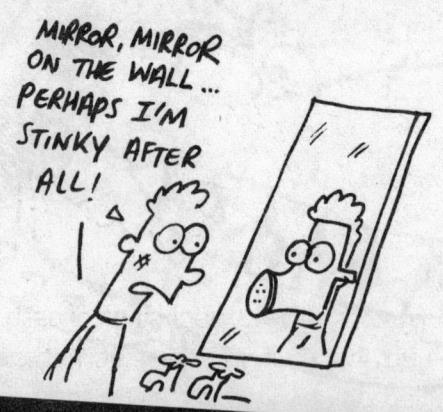

MIRROR, MIRROR ON THE WALL... PERHAPS I'M STINKY AFTER ALL!

WHAT TO DO

The best way to beat bad breath is to brush your teeth regularly – at least twice a day. Make sure you're brushing them properly and brush your tongue as well as your teeth. You can ask your dentist to show you how, if you're not sure. You are going for a check-up twice a year, aren't you? Remember that if you look after your teeth, not only will you have a healthy mouth, you'll avoid the pain of toothache!

As well as toothpaste, you can use a mouthwash and dental floss to make sure your mouth is in tip-top condition. But if you've done all this and your mouth is still a bit whiffy, don't despair. Sometimes bad breath is caused by allergies or some other illness – go and see your doctor to help sort this out.

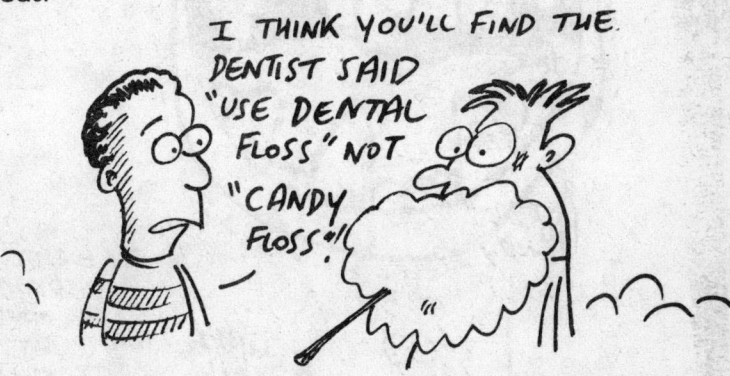

P.S. Don't forget to have a packet of breath mints or chewing gum handy if your diet sometimes includes pickled onions and cheesy crisps.

CLEAN UP YOUR CAKE HOLE

You know how it is in the mornings – you're so busy rushing to get out of the house it's easy to forget to brush your teeth. (Pee-yoo! If you had one of those mornings this morning, kindly stop breathing on the page!)

Never mind – simply cut out the horror mouth below, attach a piece of elastic, colour in using browns and yellows then place the mouth over your own. Once you've looked in the mirror you'll never be tempted to mistreat your molars again!

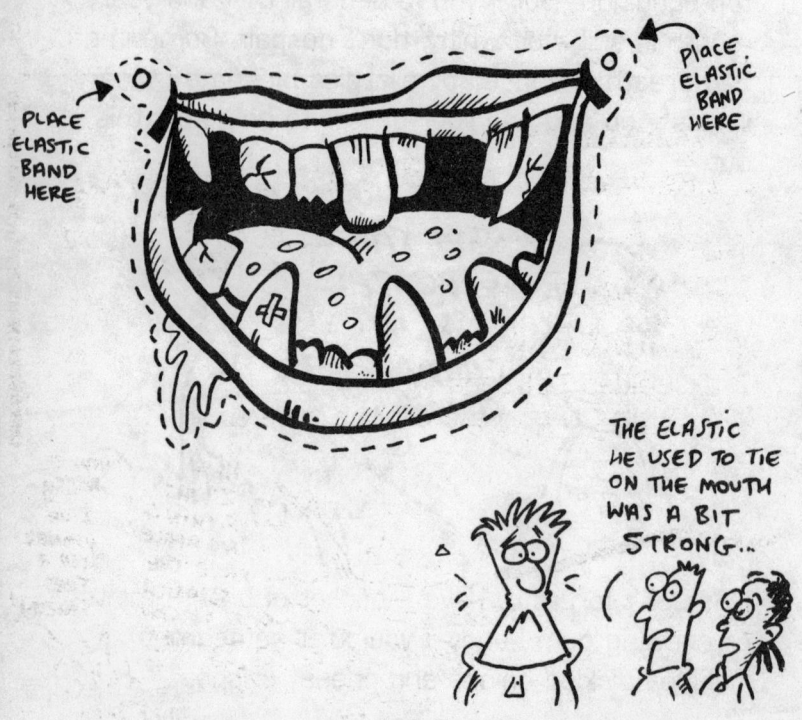

PLACE ELASTIC BAND HERE

PLACE ELASTIC BAND HERE

THE ELASTIC HE USED TO TIE ON THE MOUTH WAS A BIT STRONG...

Problems, Problems...

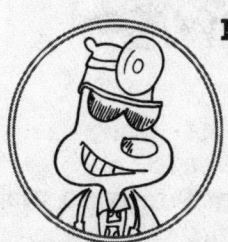

It's always good to have your medical queries answered by an expert. However, as we couldn't find one, 'Doctor' Funny has kindly agreed to step in instead.

Dear Doctor Funny
I get cold chills every night. What should I do?
Frozen, Fulham.

Dear Frozen
Stop sleeping in the fridge.

Dear Doctor Funny
I have read that an apple a day is good for my health. But everytime I pick up an apple I get a severe pain in my back.
Golden Delicious, France

Dear Golden Delicious
Try taking the apple off the tree first.

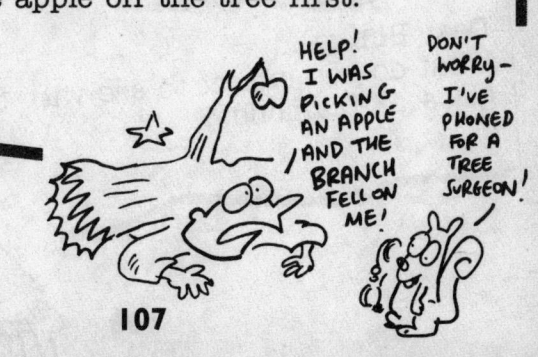

HELP! I WAS PICKING AN APPLE AND THE BRANCH FELL ON ME!

DON'T WORRY — I'VE PHONED FOR A TREE SURGEON!

Dear Doctor Funny
I woke up this morning covered in purple and green blotches. Is this catching?
Spotty, Sheffield.

Dear Spotty
We don't know – we can't get Mr Funny to pick up your letter.

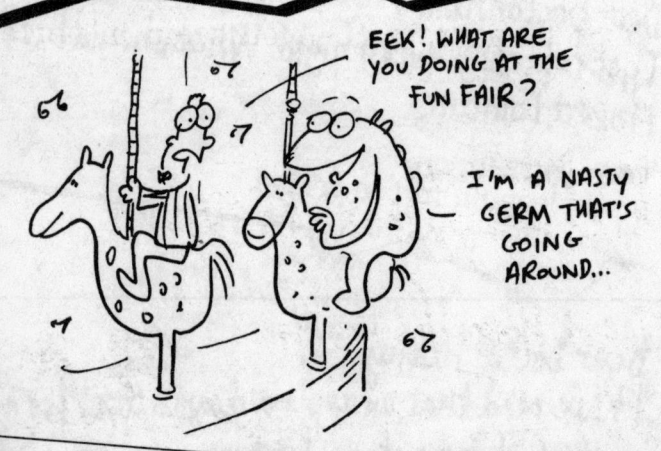

EEK! WHAT ARE YOU DOING AT THE FUN FAIR?

I'M A NASTY GERM THAT'S GOING AROUND...

Dear Doctor Funny
I recently bought some cheap glasses and now all I can see are red spots before my eyes.
Blinky, Blackburn

Dear Blinky
What do you expect to see with cheap glasses? Diamonds?

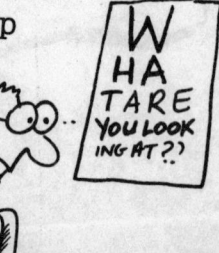

WHAT ARE YOU LOOKING AT??

Dear Doctor Funny
I have a beautiful rosy complexion, drink lots of orange juice, get lots of sunshine and am always early to bed and early to rise. What can I do?

Healthy, Harrogate

Dear Healthy
I don't understand – you seem in perfect condition to me.
Dr Funny

Dear Doctor Funny
That's what you think – I'm a Vampire.

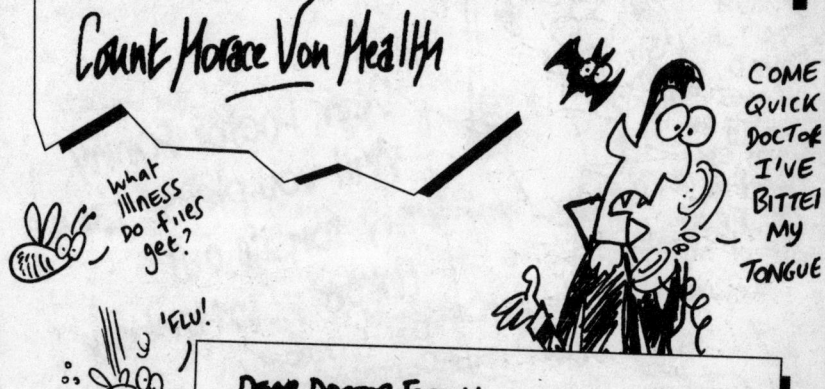

Count Horace Von Health

What illness do flies get?

'FLU!

COME QUICK DOCTOR I'VE BITTEN MY TONGUE

DEAR DOCTOR FUNNY
WHAT'S THE BEST THING TO DO ABOUT INSECT BITES?
ITCHY, IPSWICH

Dear Itchy
Stop biting insects.

109

Dear Doctor Funny
I just don't feel I'm as good as anybody else. What can I do?
Timid, Titfield

Dear Timid
Stop worrying. You are just as good as everyone else. (Mind you, anyone else would have been able to work that out for themselves.)

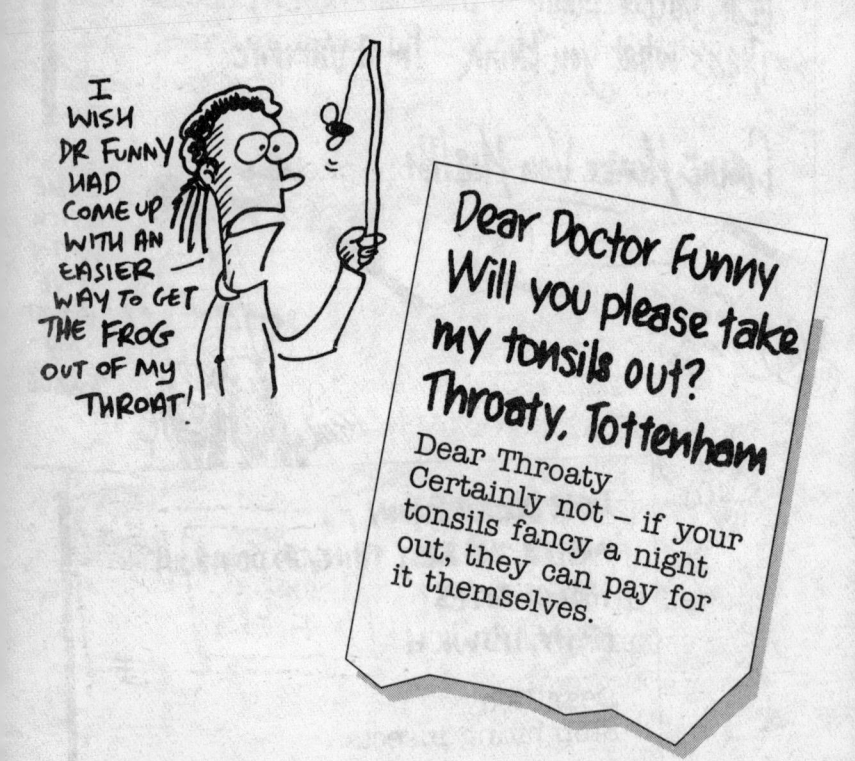

I WISH DR FUNNY HAD COME UP WITH AN EASIER WAY TO GET THE FROG OUT OF MY THROAT!

Dear Doctor Funny
Will you please take my tonsils out?
Throaty, Tottenham

Dear Throaty
Certainly not – if your tonsils fancy a night out, they can pay for it themselves.

FEE-FI-PHOBIA!

A 'phobia' is a name for a particularly bad fear of something. For some people the fear is of creepy-crawlies or thunder and lightning, for others, it's being trapped in a lift. We all have secret fears but if yours is actually stopping you from making the most of your life, it's a phobia. Most phobias can be sorted out with medical help, and until then you can take comfort in the fact that you're not the only one.

Here are some common phobias and some not so common ones that Mr Funny has recently discovered.

CLAUSTROPHOBIA
A fear of cooped-up spaces.
CLASS-TROPHOBIA
A fear of being cooped up at school. (Very common on Monday mornings.)

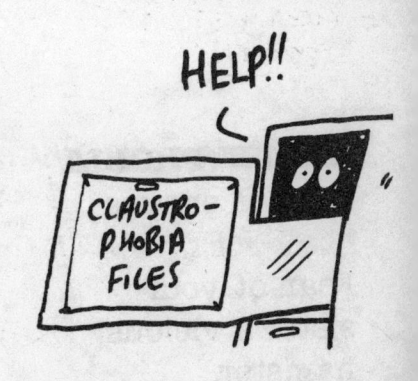

AGORAPHOBIA
Fear of wide open spaces.
AGGRO-PHOBIA
Fear of school bullies – particularly ones with wide open spaces between their ears.

ARACHNOPHOBIA
Fear of spiders.
TIE RACK-NOPHOBIA
Fear of getting something nasty from your auntie for Christmas.

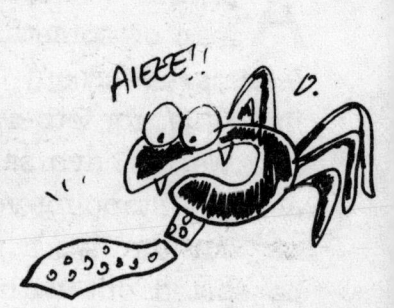

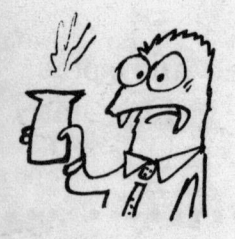

AIEEE!!

HAIR WE GO AGAIN!

HYDROPHOBIA
Fear of water.
HYDE-ROPHOBIA
Fear of accepting a glass of water from Dr Jekyll.

HERPETPHOBIA
Fear of snakes
HER-PETPHOBIA
Fear of your sister's vicious hamster.

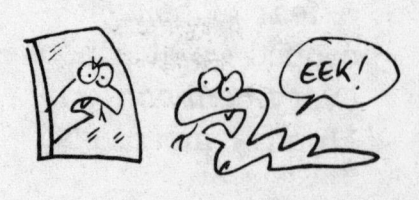

EEK!

XENOPHOBIA
Fear of foreigners.
X-FILEOPHOBIA
Fear of spooky FBI agents.

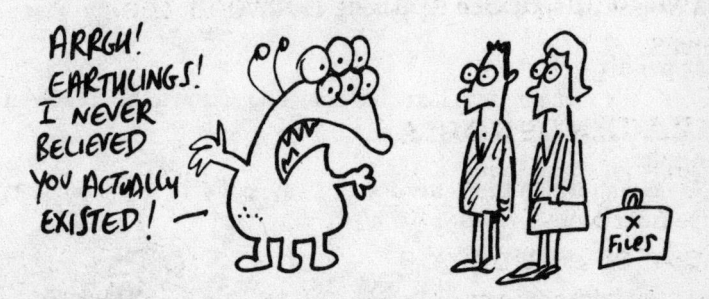

And finally...
PHOBOPHOBIA
Fear of there being something wrong with you because you're the only person who hasn't got any phobias.

MEDICAL DICTIONARY

Aerobics
Biscuits that taste like small bubbly bars of chocolate.

Ambulance
A long sharp stick used for poking an ambu.

Appendix
Sorry, the meaning was here, but someone seems to have taken it out.

Apple
Something which keeps the doctor away, but only if you jam it under the front door.

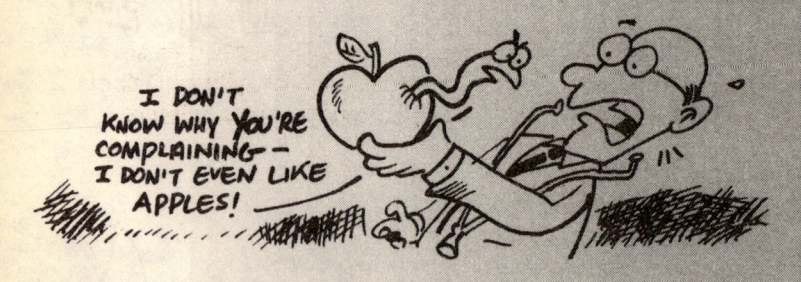

I DON'T KNOW WHY YOU'RE COMPLAINING — I DON'T EVEN LIKE APPLES!

Blood doner
A vampire's favourite kind of kebab.

Chickenpox
Small pockets on the back of a chicken's jeans.

Diet
What you do when you don't like the colour of your hair.

Doctor
Person to go to if you're sick – or being chased by a Dalek.

Hippocratic Oath
A promise doctors make never to refuse to treat a sick hippo.

Hospital
What you have to clean out of your hair after you've been spat on by a horse.

Muscles
Don't ask us, we couldn't lift the dictionary to find out.

Nurse
Person who looks after the sick. (See also *Night Nurse*: a person who looks after the sick if they're wearing suits of armour)

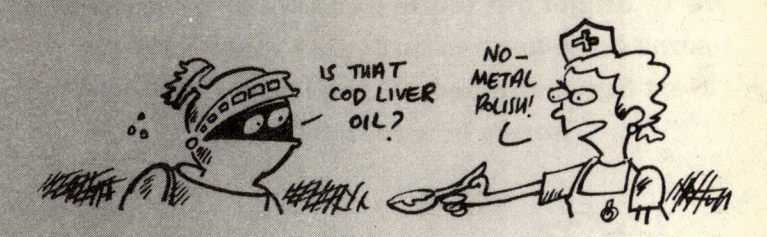

Plastic Surgery
An expensive way of changing your appearance. (See also *Wooden Surgery*: hitting yourself in the face with a plank of wood, a much cheaper way of changing your appearance.)

Skeleton
How much a skele weighs.

Undertaker
Person who looks after your body if you overdo the wooden surgery.

Underwear
Something you'd better change regularly if you want anyone to look after your body.

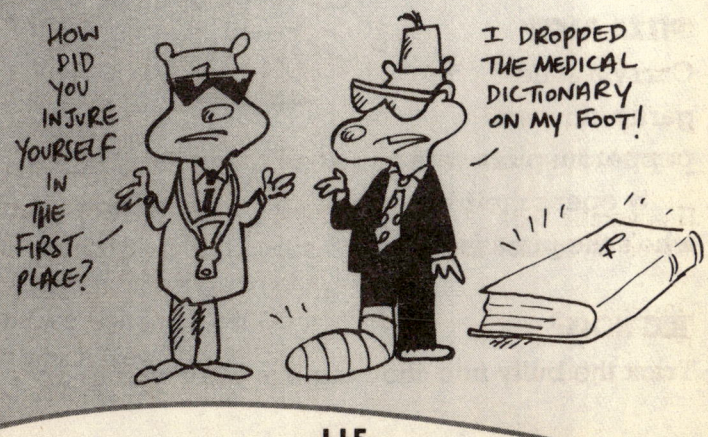

BEAT THE
BODY BULLIES

We've all got our faults – and we've all also got some bone-headed bully that picks on them. Next time somebody makes fun of your bod, here's how to fight back.

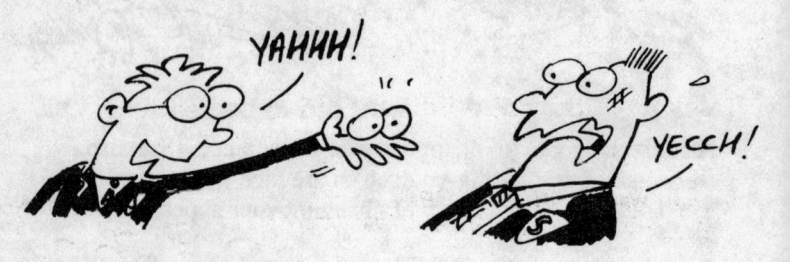

'HEY, FOUR EYES!'
Borrow a pair of glass eyes from your local optician and produce them next time someone shouts this out. They'll be sorry they ever set eyes on you.

'PIZZA FACE!'
Carry a stale garlic, tuna and pepperoni pizza with you at all times. Wait until the bully opens their big mouth and ...splatt! Now, who's the pizza face?

'BIG NOSE!'
Trick the bully into shouting this when you're on

the school trip to the zoo and standing beside the elephant house. That'll teach the bully to pick on people his own size.

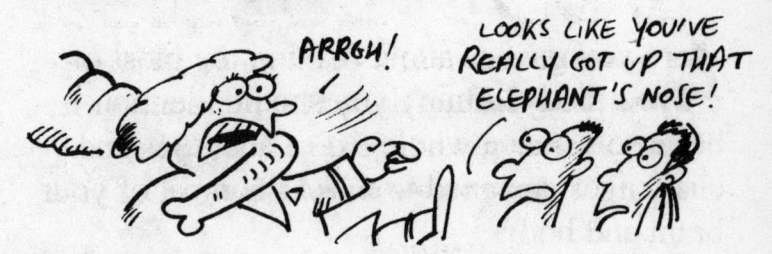

'BIG EARS!'
Tell them they're a little bit old to be reading Noddy books.

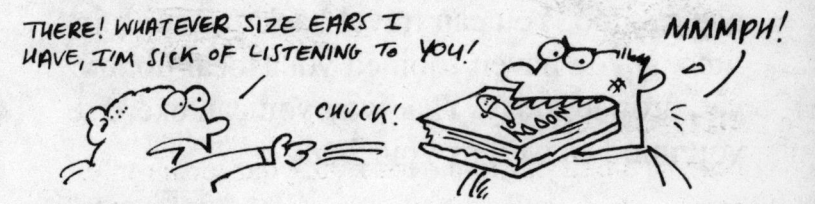

'BOG BREATH!'
Secretly alter the plumbing of the school toilet so that the flush works backwards. Make sure you're not around when the bully tries to use it as he/she may kick up a real stink.

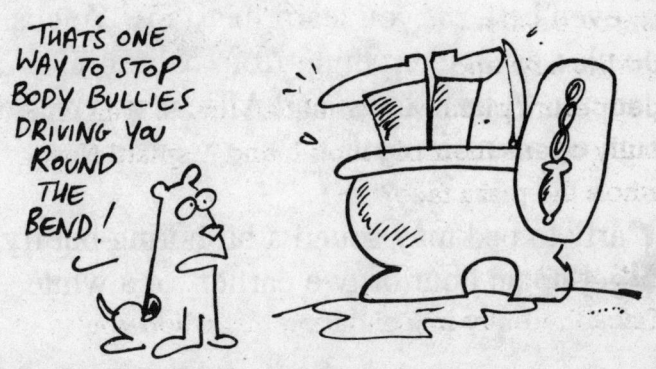

YOUR TOES TO HEAD
A-Z

Are you serious about making the most of your body? Funny you should mention it – because here's a whole list of activities and challenges designed to make the most of your brain and body.

Books are the cheapest way to travel. You can go all around the world – and to other planets, too. You can travel back and forth in time. If you haven't joined your local library yet, drop in today. That way you can exercise you mind as well as your body.

Compliment somebody! Make someone else feel good and you'll feel pretty good yourself.

Dancing is a great way of exercising – and even better if you learn the steps! You can do classes on everything from ballroom dancing to jazz, Latin and African grooves, so sign on and step out!

Early to bed may sound a bit boring but try to get up an hour or two earlier for a while.

Besides seeing a spectacular sunrise absolutely free, you might be surprised at how much you can get done before everyone else gets up and gets in your way.

Find out as much as you can about your body. It's the most important possession that you have – and it's very difficult to find a replacement.

GPs are there to help you. Never be afraid to ask your doctor (G.P. stands for General Practitioner) about anything that's worrying you health wise. Usually the problem is nowhere near as serious as you think but a few words of advice are just what the doctor ordered.

Hair plays a big part in our image, so if you fancy a change, why not go for a whole new look? After all if you don't like it, it will grow back – eventually...

Investigate a different way of living. If there are organisations for blind people, people who are deaf or people who use wheelchairs in your local area, ask if you can find out more about how these things affect the way people live. You'll discover that although not everyone's body is equipped in the same way, everybody has something interesting to teach us.

Job hunting may seem a long way away yet, but how about volunteering to help a local charity for a few hours? Besides putting your body to good use, you could make some new friends and have a lot of fun.

Knowledge is power. Learn a new fascinating fact every day (this book will give you some to start off with) and try to work it into your conversation.

Learn a musical instrument! It's a great way to keep your fingers flexible and your lungs working – although it might be a bit hard on your family's ears to start off with. There's also the possibility that you might end up being a professional musician or a rock star!

Messiest bedroom in town? Why not set aside a Saturday and give it a good clean out? Bet you'll find some brilliant stuff you thought was lost for ever. (But if you find last month's sandwiches DO NOT give way to temptation and eat them!)

Nyaah! Make the silliest face you can in the bathroom mirror. It's a lot easier to have a good day when you start with a laugh.

Older people may not get around as much as they used to, but they can certainly take you on interesting journeys. If your grandparents are still living, ask them to tell you about what they got up to when they were children. You may be just as surprised about the things that were the same as the things that were different.

Pets are great for playing with and for getting you out to exercise – unless you've got a goldfish. If your home is a bit too cooped up to keep a pet in, check if there's a city farm or animal club in your local area. You might even be able to help out at your local vet's or branch of the R.S.P.C.A. (Royal Society for the Prevention of Cruelty to Animals).

Quiet, please! Can you communicate without speaking? Set aside one Saturday as a day of silence and see if you can go about your usual activities without saying a word. Give yourself a big cheer if you can go the whole day without making a sound – it's a lot harder than you think. You could even get people to sponsor you on a 'Sponsored Silence' if you want to raise money for a charity.

Red-faced with rage? Full of frustration? Give a pillow a good duffing up. It's a great way of relieving tension and no-one gets hurt. (Do make sure there's no-one lying on the pillow before you start.)

Stun your family and friends! Secretly learn some amazing new skill – anything from juggling to playing the mouth organ. Practise in secret for six months – then in six months' time watch their jaws drop as you reveal your hidden talent!

Treat yourself every so often. It might be a favourite food, the new record by your fave group or maybe a luxurious hot bath. (Okay, we know some people might not consider bathing to be a treat!) Remember, if you're not nice to yourself, how can you expect anyone else to be?

Use your 'other hand' for a day! So if you're normally right-handed, use your left hand, and if you're left-handed, use your right. Of course, if you're ambidextrous it won't make any difference. What does 'ambidextrous' mean? Able to use both hands equally well.

Vegetarian food is good for you and these days the taste doesn't have to make you go green. Try going veggie for a week: you never know, it might grow on you!

Water is good for your body, both inside and outside. It's never too late to learn to swim – if you can't yet, sign up for classes at your local pool. If you can, how about starting to learn about life-saving or water safety? Baywatch, here you come!

Xpecting us to be stumped by this letter? No way. Grab a pencil and the crossword in today's newspaper and test your word power.

You have the only body of its kind in the world and there's never going to be one like it again. So take care of it, make the most of it. And one other thing...

Zee you in the next **Seriously Funny Guide!!!**

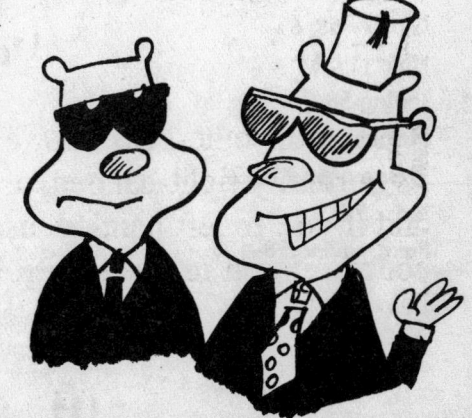

Index of serious body bits

Acne 72, 73
Age (fun facts) 84–89
Bad breath 104, 105
Blues/depression 90, 91
Body (fun facts) 96, 97
Body language 52–55
Body odour (B.O.) 14, 15
Body shapes 11, 12
Cartilage 56
Childline 91
Colour blindness 75
Dancing 118
Dandruff 50, 51
Death (fun facts) 36–38
Dehydration 43
Dentist 105
Doctor (G.P.) 28, 43, 51, 73, 105, 119
Ectomorph 11, 12
Endomorph 11, 12
Face (fun facts) 74, 75
Food (fun facts) 16, 17
Glasses 68, 69
Hair 119, 51
Jet lag 58
Melanin 42
Mesomorph 11, 12
Nose 74
Palmreading 98–100

ARRGH! I'M ALLERGIC TO THE INDEX!

ITCH!

BLOTCH!

Phobias 111–113
    Agoraphobia 112
    Arachnophobia 112
    Claustrophobia 111
    Herpetphobia 113
    Hydrophobia 112
    Xenophobia 113
Sebum 72
Seriously Funny Workout, The 21-29
    Be a Desk Dynamo 28, 29
    Face Up To It 27
    Jump To It 25
    Toe Touches 23
    Totally Arm-azing 26
    Waist To Go 24
    Warming Up 21
Scalp 51
Sleep facts 56-58
Sleepwalking 57
Snoring 57
Spots 72, 73
Sunburn 42, 43
Sweating 14, 15
Swimming 123
Tanning 42
Teeth 74, 75, 105
Vegetarianism 123

HAVE YOU LOOKED UP YOUR PHOBIA IN THE SERIOUSLY FUNNY GUIDE'S INDEX?

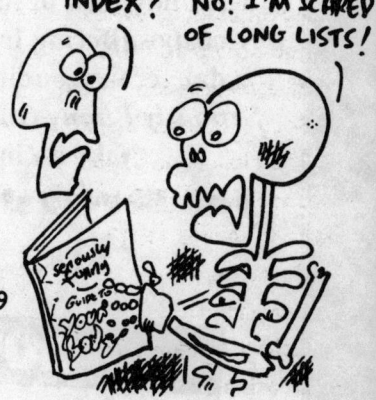

NO! I'M SCARED OF LONG LISTS!

WHERE'S THE CARTOON ABOUT SWEATING?

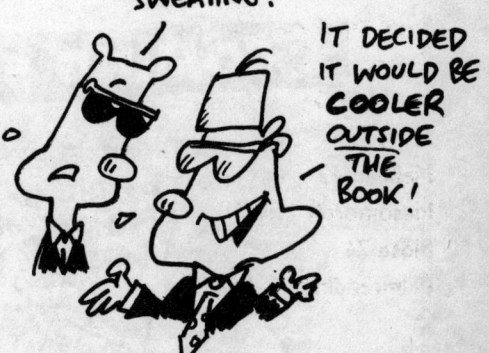

IT DECIDED IT WOULD BE COOLER OUTSIDE THE BOOK!

PRESCRIPTION

So you're suffering from depression, a heavy heart and lack of funny-bone exercise? You're obviously suffering from 'Seriofunniconclusivitus' – a dangerous condition caused by finishing your *Seriously Funny Guide*. Dr Funny suggests you take an immediate dose of:

The Seriously Funny Guide to the Movies

OUT NOW

If this doesn't work, try:

The Seriously Funny Guide to Pets

The Seriously Funny Guide to Spooky Stuff

COMING SOON

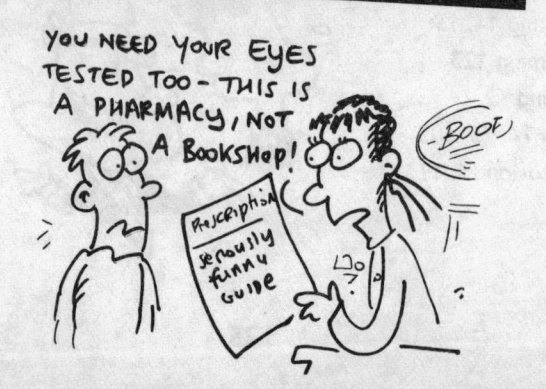

YOU NEED YOUR EYES TESTED TOO - THIS IS A PHARMACY, NOT A BOOKSHOP!

BOO!

PRESCRIPTION
Seriously Funny Guide